THE CALL
AND THE ANSWER

Laurence Binyon was born in Lancaster in 1869. He was an eminent poet and art historian, with a particular interest in Chinese and Japanese painting. He worked at the British Museum for forty years, latterly as Keeper of Prints and Drawings. In 1933 he succeeded TS Eliot as the Norton Professor of Poetry at Harvard University. Binyon was over-age for military service when war broke out in 1914, but volunteered as a medical orderly, serving in the 'English hospital' for French soldiers at Arc-en-Barrois, near Verdun. In 1917 he toured the battlefields and hospitals of France at the request of the British Red Cross. He died in 1943.

THE CALL
AND THE ANSWER

LAURENCE BINYON

First published as *For Dauntless France* in Great Britain in 1918 by Hodder and Stoughton. This slightly abridged version first published in Great Britain in 2018 as *The Call and the Answer* by Dare-Gale Press.

Dare-Gale Press, 15-17 Middle Street, Brighton BN1 1AL

www.daregale.com

The publisher is grateful to the Society of Authors as the Literary Representative of the Estate of Laurence Binyon.

Introduction © Llorenç O'Prey 2018
Front cover: VAD recruitment poster by Joyce Dennys (1915) reproduced with permission of Curtis Brown Group Ltd, London, on behalf of the beneficiaries of the estate of Joyce Dennys. Copyright © Joyce Dennys 1917. Image © Imperial War Museums (Art.IWM PST 3268)

ISBN 9780993331121

Printed By TJ International, Padstow

CONTENTS

Introduction 7

The Witnesses 10

PART I – THE CALL AND THE ANSWER

The Scene Surveyed 15

A Day's Work at the Office of the *Comité Britannique* 31

British Nurses in France: The French Flag Nursing Corps 47

PART II – THE RECORD

The Convoys:

    The First Year 57

    Verdun 99

    And After 117

The Hospitals:

    Hospital Supply Depots: And the French War

    Emergency Fund 133

    The Story of the Hospitals 146

    The Day of an Orderly 199

The Canteens 221

Relief Work in the Devastated Zones 252

PART III – IMPRESSIONS

On the Front in Champagne 273

A Canteen in the Forest 279

Hospitals in and about Paris 285

Ruins and Refugees   293
Lyons and Nevers   304
In the Vosges   311
Some Canteens in the War Zone   319
Verdun to Chalons   328
In the Midi   340
A Maternity Hospital   355
A Thought for the Future   361

INTRODUCTION

At the outbreak of war in 1914 one of the most urgent questions to be addressed was how to prepare for the very large number of casualties which were expected to be a feature of modern, industrialised warfare – in other words, how to care for wounded or sick soldiers on a scale previously unimagined. The knowledge that emergency medical support was available on the battlefield would be essential to maintain the morale of troops held in situations of intense and prolonged hardship and danger. Neither Britain nor France was fully prepared for such a situation and would clearly need to call upon a great number of civilian volunteers to provide the services needed. Just as many young men were drawn by the national call to arms, thousands of men and women responded willingly to an urgent call to serve in the interests of saving life. They volunteered with the numerous medical and voluntary aid organisations which grew rapidly in response to the needs of soldiers wounded in battle, including the British Red Cross and the Voluntary Aid Detachments (VADs).

Laurence Binyon was one such volunteer, taking time from his work as a curator at the British Museum to serve as a medical orderly in France. Binyon is perhaps best remembered for writing the four lines of poetry that are carved onto countless war memorials and that today are still recited at every Service of Remembrance:

They shall grow not old, as we that are left grow old:
Age shall not weary them, nor the years condemn.
At the going down of the sun and in the morning
We will remember them.

Binyon wrote 'For the Fallen' in September 1914, in response to the losses sustained by the British Expeditionary Force at the Battle of Mons and the Battle of Marne, and almost as if foreseeing the carnage that was to follow. The poem's tender and reflexive tone expressed both a public sense of grief for a nation traumatised by loss, and helped to meet a private need for consolation.

By 1914 Binyon had established a reputation as a distinguished art historian and accomplished poet. He was forty-five years old and therefore over-age for the Army, but like a great many others he felt a strong sense of duty to support the war effort in some way. For such a person, he wrote, 'there was one great field of opportunity: helping the wounded.' In July 1915 he used his annual leave to volunteer as an *ambulancier* and medical orderly at the *Hôpital Temporaire* at Arc-en-Barrois in the Haute-Marne, where the writer John Masefield and painter Henry Tonks also volunteered in a similar role. Binyon returned again in the summer of 1916 to help treat soldiers injured in the Battle of Verdun.

Binyon's war experiences affected him profoundly. He was shocked by the terrible 'wasting and maiming' he witnessed at Arc-en-Barrois and by the suffering he saw for himself on visits to many other hospitals across France. The poems he wrote once he got to the Front strike a more personal and bitter note than 'For the Fallen'. At Arc-en-Barrois he developed close friendships with many of the '*Poilus*', the ordinary French soldiers whom he came to admire – the 'lads in the loose blue' he describes in his poem 'The Witnesses', included here.

In 1917 Binyon was asked by the British Red Cross Society to write an account of British volunteer aid efforts in support of 'the French wounded and victims of the war'. Originally published in 1918 as *For Dauntless France*, the resulting book provided a detailed account of the diverse range of activities and support offered to the French by British private individuals and organisations. This centenary edition is slightly abridged in omitting the appendices and other material of a more statistical nature and takes its title 'The Call and the Answer' from Part One.

Binyon's research for the book entailed visiting numerous hospitals, ambulance stations and field canteens across France, including well-known operations such as the Millicent Sutherland Ambulance (page 148) and the field hospital on the Somme, whose benefactor and *Directrice* was the poet Mary Borden (pages 182-3). He interviewed the men and women volunteers he met there and drew on his own experiences which he describes in detail in the chapter 'The Day of an Orderly'. Binyon's survey gives both a sense of scale of the efforts, as well as a vivid and sympathetic account of the experiences of individual volunteers and the wounded soldiers who they helped.

The war exacted a profound toll on those who were touched by it. From the extremes of violence and suffering, however, emerged acts of great compassion and humanity. As with 'For the Fallen', Binyon's account of volunteer aid workers on the Western Front is at once sombre and hopeful. It highlights the scale of the suffering, alongside the heroism and fortitude of the many volunteers who contributed to its alleviation, often under conditions of great hardhip and personal risk to themselves.

Llorenç O'Prey

The Witnesses

I

Lads in the loose blue,
Crutched, with limping feet,
With bandaged arm, that roam
To-day the bustling street,

You humble us with your gaze,
Calm, confiding, clear;
You humble us with a smile
That says nothing but cheer.

Our souls are scarred with you!
Yet, though we suffered all
You have suffered, all were vain
To atone, or to recall

The robbed future, or build
The maimed body again
Whole, or ever efface
What men have done to men.

II

Each body of straight youth,
Strong, shapely, and marred,
Shines as out of a cloud
Of storm and splintered shard,

Of chaos, torture, blood,
Fire, thunder, and stench:
And the savage shattering noise
Of churned and shaken trench

Echoes through myriad hearts
In the dumb lands behind; –
Silent wailing, and bitter
Tears of the world's mind!

You stand upon each threshold
Without complaint. – What pen
Dares to write half the deeds
That men have done to men?

III
Must we be humbled more?
Peace, whose olive seems
A tree of hope and heaven,
Of answered prayers and dreams,

Peace has her own hid wounds;
She also grinds and maims.
And must we bear and share
Those old continued shames?

Not only the body's waste
But the mind's captivities –
Crippled, sore, and starved –
The ignorant victories

Of the visionless, who serve
No cause, and fight no foe!
Is a cruelty less sure
Because its ways are slow?

Now we have eyes to see.
Shall we not use them then?
These bright wounds witness
What men may do to men.

PART I

THE CALL AND THE ANSWER

THE SCENE SURVEYED

Imagine yourself, at any time these three years, transported to some aerial vantage-point above the regions of Western Europe.

There beneath you lie the mapped plains of France, melting northward in the mists of the Channel. Toward the east, sombre patches mark the rolling forests of the Ardennes. Like a barrier to the featureless Chalons plain, rises the long, wooded chine of the Argonne. The shining of rivers is visible: Marne and Aube and Aisne, Sambre and Meuse and Moselle. Far off, toward the coast, is the black country of pits and chimneys: and following the frontier southward you might discern the hills that defend Verdun, the swellings of the Vosges, the Rhine in its valley beyond them, and a distance heaping itself into the snowy Alps.

Like the disembodied aerial spectator of Mr. Hardy's *Dynasts*, you look down on a world at war. Europe is busy with the same martial ferment, it is scarred with the same frequency of ravage and misery on its surface as a hundred odd years ago.

Yet with a difference. Then, the picture might have seemed that of Napoleon's glittering and voracious armies preying on more or less passive populations, as they turned this way and that in their vast 'sheep-worry of Europe.' But now, if ordinary sight could for a moment be transcended and the divining power of imagination translated into physical sense, so that what is invisible in men's activity became visible, you would be aware of a scene of grandeur, epical in its significance; a scene of human effort on a scale unparalleled since the world began. You would be aware of whole nations pouring their last energy into a conflict which exacts something from each man and woman and child, however removed from the actual battle, and from millions has exacted everything. It is a challenge that knocks on every door; that takes its toll not only of flesh and blood, and food and money, but of dear illusions, and even of rooted faiths. It dissolves inveterate customs in a day. It crumbles old systems and great empires from within. Far from being passive, these populations – how vastly increased by a century's growth! – combine in a willed effort like that of a single wrestler, hardly conceivable in its prolonged intensity. We need not fable, in the old Homeric way, the presence of gods of battle, succouring and inspiring mortal man, for you would be aware of Ideas, terrible and inexorable powers, ranged on either side, and compelling weak flesh to endure unendurable things.

To the eye there would appear those mapped plains and undulations of Eastern France; cities famed in history since the twilight of the early Middle Ages; rivers and intersecting roads; the mesh of railways and canals. But you would also become conscious that on road and rail there was a movement of men and arms directed eastwards, increasing in density as it approaches a certain irregular line, like a scar, that can be followed from the sand-dunes of the Flanders coasts to the pines of the Jura. Groups, masses, battalions; cars, lorries, trucks, machines; it is like the orderly streaming of ants with their burdens, an intricate order moving in the one direction; but always it ends in that irregular scarred line, where suddenly the men disappear, and guns – terrible, untiring, impersonal – seem to usurp their places.

You would remark that these streams of moving figures,

above a certain point, are in uniform that makes a tawny smudge on the landscape; below that point it is smudges of misty blue that tell of moving battalions.

That scarred line, from Yser to Jura, attracts like a magnet; it sucks up like a sponge. All Europe, and much more than Europe, is conscious of it. Not a hamlet by the Atlantic or the remote Pyrenees – not a village in the British Isles but has a vision of it; and far away in the South Seas and beyond the North Atlantic it is the same. To it men and women are sending, sending, sending. They have sent sons and brothers, lovers and husbands. They have sent arms and munitions. They are sending letters and little gifts. Those that have nothing send their thoughts and their fears. Could we use that other vision of the mind, we might see those thoughts, prayers, curses, apprehensions, hopes and passionate desires flying in that one direction like the birds that fill the sky at the time of their migration. But we should also see, pressing thither, streams of embodied human energy – passion and calculation alike translated into active force and absorbed into the momentum of a single will.

And these animated energies, collected and deepened in pressure and volume as they approach the battle-front, pour forward ceaselessly to meet an opposing tide that draws its strength from the German lands beyond. The two vast tides clash in a conflict that never ends, that never sleeps; that dies down to intervals of seeming quiet, but wakes again to double and triple fury. And all along that line the earth is blotched, pounded, pitted, scorched. The trees are splintered stumps. It is a landscape that is to the natural green and brown like the face of an idiot among the healthy and bright-eyed. An insane landscape, smelling of evil. It resounds with all the noises of chaos. By night it alternates thick gloom with sudden and sinister illumination. Yet the larks go up in the dawns and sing above the cannonade.

Here is a whole nation that presses and thrusts against the obstinate force of another nation. And it might even seem as if the very soil of France laboured and sacrificed itself in an identity of cause and purpose, just as the body's deep instinct is to expel a poisoning evil that has fixed on it. For it is French soil the Germans hold, and use and abuse at will.

That confluence and concentration of prodigious effort has one end: to destroy. It feeds an inconceivable hunger that is never satisfied; the hunger of the guns.

Yet look a little longer. You will see another activity revealed, less strong, less imposing, less vehement, but as constant, though moving in the opposite direction.

From that scarred line which attracts to itself so enormous a stream of human effort directed deathwards, there flows also back another stream of effort directed lifewards.

Sometimes a mere trickle; but at other times, after the bombardments and assaults, it swells suddenly like a river in spate. But no, let us eschew metaphors like these. They are callous, they blunt our senses, they blur the reality; they are too like that talk of 'human material' that the German High Command affects, with its proud military science and its bestial contempt of human kind. Enough of metaphors, though we fly to them for help because our minds are overwhelmed by the weights of uncalculated numbers. Let us fix our minds on the truth that of all these thousands and hundreds of thousands – material shovelled into the trenches as good 'stopping-stuff,' let Germans call them if they will – each one is a single soul, a single body, sensitive to pain as you or I. Each one that returns from those trenches is a man returning from hell.

A train, badged with the Red Cross, crawls over the landscape, moving westward. It is a peaceful landscape on which the twilight has descended; a great green plain rising into ridge and woody plateau. The guns of the French front are still audible at times, but only as a faint shock upon the ear.

Let us assume the privilege of the aerial spectator, and descend to closer quarters.

The train comes ever so slowly to a stop at a little station by the roadside. You can see through the windows French soldiers in their grey-blue uniform, bandaged about the head or arm, with their heads leant back on the partitions or on each other's shoulders, in attitudes of animal weariness and stupor. A few perhaps, more lightly wounded, will look out of the window, exchange a word with a comrade, wonder how far the train has brought them, light and puff at a cigarette. But all are very weary.

These are the sitting cases. The other half of the train is closed and dark. But now the orderlies begin to bring out the *couchés* on their stretchers, and lay them side by side on the platform. The doctor in charge of the train is there, directing and giving orders: and to him come, saluting, those who are to receive the wounded and take them off to hospital. A row of grey motor ambulances waits outside the station.

But why are these others in English khaki? They are English plainly, by their looks and figures: and here and there a wounded Frenchman looks up with just a little curiosity overcoming his vast fatigue as he hears the English voices.

In a few minutes the train will have crept away into the dusk, to discharge its burden by degrees at one station after another. But already the men on the stretchers have been given a drink, and wrapped in a warm blanket. The English doctor asks each where his wound is, and rapidly examines the writing on the label tied to his tunic. A red label means a severe wound; a blue label, a less severe wound, though often still serious. The slightly wounded have a white label; but these come rarely this way.

The ambulances are quickly filled, and they glide off.

Soon they will be arriving at the hospital, probably a château or lycée or disused convent converted to this use for the war. Each will be allotted to a ward, and quickly washed and put to bed by English nurses. The stained uniform, helmet, boots, and pathetic little belongings of the soldier are neatly tied up, packed and ticketed; and at last he gets to his good sleep, no longer jolted by wheels beneath him.

For a week, for a month, probably for many weeks or many months, these Frenchmen will be living under the care of British surgeons, with British nurses dressing their wounds, talking to them of their homes and families, helping their first crippled steps, cheering on their recovery – in a word, making friends of them.

For we have chanced upon a unit of one of those improvisations of the war, which, from scattered efforts and casual beginnings, have grown to surprising dimensions. These hospitals where the British tend the French are scattered about France; you will find them in Normandy and Brittany as well as in the departments of the East, in Meuse, and Oise, and Haute Marne; on the Mediterranean and in the central provinces. And besides these British hospitals there are in numbers of the French hospitals, English, Scottish, and Irish women working as nurses.

But the hospitals are only one side of this work that Britain, out of her desire to help, has done in France. It is quite likely that some of those wounded we have seen in the Red Cross train were carried from the first-aid post at the front by English ambulances, driven by English volunteers. Fully equipped sections of these ambulances serve on the French front. Each convoy – and there are some sixteen of them – contains twenty or more motor ambulances, and each serves a division of the French Army.

And besides the hospitals and the convoys, there are some fifty canteens scattered up and down the country, at stations and barracks and rest-camps, where English ladies serve free refreshments to the tired soldiers on their way to or from the trenches, and give them entertainments. At one of these canteens as many as fifteen thousand soldiers have been served with drink and cigarettes in a single day.

This activity is relatively only a small part of the vast ramified work of the French Red Cross; but what does it mean? It means that hundreds of thousands of wounded French soldiers have passed through friendly British hands – carried on ambulances, refreshed at canteens, or actually nursed and doctored. And of these there will be many thousands who have passed long weeks and months with English men and women in familiar acquaintance.

In those sad regions, the regions of devastation, you will find more English people, working for the Society of Friends, who have helped to build huts for the homeless refugees, to give them clothing and seeds to sow the land with, and to persuade them out of their first apathy and despair.

If we emphasise the fact that the great majority of these workers are volunteers, who in many cases give more than their time and their services, it is because it is right to point out that what we have done has been a spontaneous thing, a gesture of homage and friendship for the France we admire. In that spirit it was offered; in that spirit it was accepted.

During that long time when our new armies were preparing, and while the French were supporting, along so immense a front, the whole brunt and burden of the Western War, how many of us in England were impatient and restless! What a glorious relief it was to those who could engage in this work and feel that in some small way they were helping heroic France! It was a privilege and a joy.

When all these workers have returned to their homes in Britain, they will testify to what they have seen and known.

They will have learnt that Paris is not France, and that the tourist of other days but rarely came into touch with the true French nature, with France herself. They will grow to understand how fine is the texture of human qualities and human resources which underlie French history, French art and civilisation, and which have made the French so great and renowned a people. One and all of our workers have come to feel an extraordinary respect and love for the simple Poilu. They have seen him in the time of his trial and suffering. They will tell how uncomplaining he is, how cheerful in hard conditions; how amenable, how innately courteous; how ready to do all and bear all for the sake of his own France.

And all those soldiers of France, when they too have returned to their homes, scattered over every province from the Channel to the Mediterranean, from the Pyrenees to

Calais Sands, what will they say of the English?

It is not for us to answer. But at least, when the name of England is spoken among them, it will not be an abstraction distilled from newspaper articles that floats before their minds, vague and alien, but certain human faces which they remember, certain men and women who worked hard and did kind things because they liked to do them.

We all remember the earthquake suddenness – for the general public at all events – of the war's explosion. Everyone felt the terrible urgency of the moment. It seemed as if in six months, in six weeks even, all might be lost. The necessity of doing something cried to our hearts night and day: but what could be done? Young and fit men could enrol in the great army that England was preparing; but what could the others do, the older men and the women? Happy then were those who were in any fashion prepared for the crisis and occasion. There was one great field of opportunity: helping the wounded. It was soon foreseen that the war, though at the outset sanguinely expected to be over in a few months, would be fought on a scale surpassing history or legend. And the murderous machinery of modern warfare promised also casualties never paralleled. It so happened that England, so far less prepared for a Continental campaign than France, excelled in one respect, in the provision of trained nurses for the wounded. Since the days of Florence Nightingale, public opinion had been brought to regard nursing as a serious and noble profession requiring an arduous training; and the number of women who had taken up this profession was very great. In France, before the separation of Church and State, nursing was almost entirely in the hands of the nuns. The nuns left

France, and left a gap which could not be filled up at once. The profession of nursing, against which a prejudice still lingered, had only begun to be taken up seriously when war broke out. The war has changed these conditions; but in the early autumn of 1914 France was in great and immediate need, and we in Britain counted ourselves fortunate that in this way we had means to aid her. We were the more able to help, because at that time the service of voluntary units was not desired by our own military authorities.

Societies of old standing; societies hastily formed for the purpose; individuals, groups of friends, all were urgent with offers of funds, stores, and personal service.

In July of that year all Britain had been hanging on the horror of civil war in Ireland; and for a long time, the campaign for Women's Suffrage had absorbed the most feverish energies. In a twinkling Germany transformed the scene! The Women Suffragists of Scotland now turned their admirable organisation to the war's use, giving hospitals and staffs to France, and also to Serbia; in Ulster the North Tyrone Volunteers, having their Medical Corps fully equipped, placed it at the service of the French. These were typical examples of the way in which existing material and trained skill were utilised forthwith. But from all sides came the offers of help. All over these islands there rose, like an immense tide, a volume of goodwill, eager to serve and to be used. How was this great tide to be guided through orderly channels so as beneficially to reach the wounded men whom we longed to succour, and who were the sole object of these offers? That is the story we have to tell.

There are three Red Cross Societies in France: *La Société de Secours aux Blessés Militaires*, the *Association des Dames*

Françaises, and the *Union des Femmes de France*. The last-named alone of these Societies had a committee in London, a committee already established for a long time before the war: and this committee during the first months was eminently useful. But Monsieur Paul Cambon, the French Ambassador, soon perceived that a special organisation was necessary to deal with all the offers of help made to the Embassy and to co-ordinate and expedite the various units accepted by the French. He therefore called into being the *Comité de Londres* or London Committee, now known as the *Comité Britannique* or British Committee, of the French Red Cross. The wife of the Military Attaché became *Présidente*: H.M. Queen Alexandra graciously consented to become Patroness of the *Comité d'Honneur*, which contains a number of distinguished and influential names. Monsieur Cambon and the members of the French Embassy have given the committee their cordial support. Offices were found at 25 Knightsbridge, afterwards removed to No. 9. It is to Monsieur Cambon's prescience and the timely creation, towards the close of 1914, of this committee that there has been so little overlapping or waste in a work which, fed from the most diverse sources, was rapidly to grow to great dimensions.

What did this work consist of? On one side were the French needs; here of a hospital staff, there of a convoy of motor-ambulances; medical stores, drugs, dressings, wanted all the more because the chief manufacturing districts of France passed with the first invasion into the German hands. There were hospitals which needed an addition to their staff of nurses, or support, in poor districts, for beds. On the other side were the offers of help from Britain: funds, stores, clothing, cars, surgeons, nurses, ambulance drivers, orderlies. The essential function of the London Committee was to utilise the gift or service offered so as best to satisfy each particular need that arose.

Collection, allocation, and distribution of funds and material gifts have occupied one department of the committee exclusively.

To deal with stores is a comparatively simple matter. But when it is a question of men and women offering their services in time of war, it becomes complex. Nothing and no one can be taken for granted. And here the co-operation of the British Red Cross Society and the Order of St. John of Jerusalem proved an invaluable help. The Anglo-French Committee (Since the end of 1917 united with the *Comité Britannique*) of these joint societies has worked throughout in close accord with the *Comité de Londres*. It was important to ensure that only the best workers should go to France; and in the scrutiny of credentials and issue of certificates to British workers, the Anglo-French Committee has done the greatest service.

At the beginning of the war the regulations affecting the entry of British subjects into France were not strict. Several units found their way over to help the French wounded; and they performed pioneer work under the most difficult conditions. But before long it was seen that more stringent regulations were necessary; and many a would-be Red Cross worker, or group of workers, who had contemplated rushing to the aid of the heroic French wounded, found themselves held up and unable to proceed till after long delays.

The British Red Cross Society authorised workers to assist the wounded of our own army, and, under the sanction of the War Office, investigated their credentials. But when it was a case of British workers wanting to serve in the French war zone, there were obvious difficulties. Unless a strict examination of each person's trustworthiness were made, it was an opportunity for the most undesirable and dangerous people to insinuate themselves among the French forces.

The British Red Cross Society and the Order of St. John, amalgamated in October 1914, were therefore asked by the War Office to undertake this task of sifting the credentials of all British applicants for Red Cross work with the French. The joint societies agreed. They delegated the work to a sub-committee, known as the Anglo-French Hospitals Committee, which was interested in the work of certain units then being formed for service with the French wounded, and which we have already mentioned.

Early in 1915 a certificate began to be issued by this committee to all would-be workers who had passed its scrutiny.

The *Comité de Londres*, always in close touch with the French Embassy and French War Office, welcomed the appearance of this Anglo-French certificate, since the stringent conditions under which it was issued did all that was possible to exclude any abuse of the Red Cross, and guaranteed that the services of qualified workers only were placed at the disposal of the French. The *Comité de Londres* worked hand in hand with the Anglo-French Committee in the selection of British personnel; and it has also given facilities for allied and neutral workers, all of whom pass through the office at 9 Knightsbridge.

It was soon decided that a special uniform was necessary, and a uniform of khaki, with blue on the collar and cuffs, was agreed on between the British and French War Offices; and men who held the Anglo-French certificate were authorised to wear it.

And who were these thousands of men and women who have gone out from these islands to work for the wounded of France?

First we must name the surgeons.

These have gone out, mostly as volunteers, to serve for varying periods. Many have given what would in other years have been their holidays. They have made sacrifices both of time and of money, all the more generous when it is remembered how exacting and heavy were the demands on them at home.

Then there are the nurses.

Who, that has seen them at work, has not admired their skill, their resource, their patient deftness? They have behind them a hard and splendid training, which ensures that only enthusiasts for the vocation become fully qualified nurses. Very few had experience of war, and the wounds a modern war produces; therefore their interests were all the more engaged. But it is not only their own work that has been invaluable, it is the training they have given to others less skilled. For under the nurses or sisters work the VAD probationers.

Truly the VADs have become a legend of the war. In those days that now seem so strangely divided from us, the days before the war, the British Red Cross Society occupied itself in forming Voluntary Aid Detachments in local centres; these detachments were to help our sol-diers in case of armed invasion by an enemy. The specific aim was to fill the gap in the Territorial Medical Service between the Clearing Hospital and the Base. The object seemed perhaps remote and academic in those days: but it was a providential instinct apparently which prompted the formation of these detachments. The Red Cross Society itself, as Sir Frederick Treves has reminded us – quartered in three small rooms in Victoria Street – owned in July 1914 not a single ambulance, 'could not provide a single bed, had not even a storeroom of its own, nor any supplies at its disposal.' To what a vast organisation has it grown in three years! And what wonder-workers have been the VADs!

At first there was in the professional world an apprehension that hospitals might be filled with quite untrained women donning the Red Cross, and that the unfortunate experiences of the Boer War might be repeated. But during the five years before the war, the original VADs had worked hard and well, and a number of women had trained themselves in discipline and drill, had learnt nursing and sanitation, as well as cooking, and other smaller arts by the way. There was therefore, when war began, an organisation ready to absorb the recruits that flocked to it; there were a standard and a tradition to maintain.

The VADs, however, would be the first to acknowledge how much they owe to the fully trained nurses under whom they work. In the hospitals for the French soldiers, the value of their work has been enhanced by the fact that practically all of them speak French – many of them extremely well. Bred in gentle homes, they have shrunk from no task, however distasteful or repulsive. Yet among them are girls who, before the war, or at its outset, protested that nothing would induce them to face the wounds and horrors of a hospital.

'The VADs are undoubtedly the surprise. They are splendid, and as probationers under trained nurses in a ward, nothing that I can say is good enough for them.' So writes a surgeon in his report.

The ambulance drivers of the British Convoys with the French are many of them gentleman-volunteers, mostly over military age, who often give an ambulance car as well as drive it. They are attached to the French army, receive the French soldier's rations; they pass a great part of their time in dug-outs, and work under fire. Besides these volunteers there are a certain number of paid drivers.

In the hospitals conditions vary; some have English volunteers as chauffeurs or as orderlies. And there are a number of ladies who work as secretaries, as cooks, and in various household capacities.

It is ladies also who manage as well as maintain the canteens, where the hours are often long and the labour hard.

But let not the reader, because we are here concerned solely with this British effort, forget for a moment the immense activities of the three great Societies of the Red Cross in France, to which this effort was, of course, but supplementary. The Societies, with the experience of 1870 behind them, had been long prepared for the eventuality of war, and (with branches in every town) could at once place many thousands of beds at the disposal of the *Service de Santé* – though, as we shall see, the scale of the war and its suddenness, created a pressure beyond anticipation or belief. And if France had not the resources in professional nursing enjoyed by Britain, the French Red Cross workers, corresponding to our VADs, were ready at the outbreak of war in great numbers, each with several months of training. They have done a wonderful work.

A DAY'S WORK

AT THE OFFICE OF THE *COMITÉ BRITANNIQUE*

How is the reader to be given an at all sufficient notion or lively picture of the work of the *Comité Britannique*?

One normally thinks of a committee as meeting from time to time round a table, going through an agenda paper, instructing its secretary and sub-committees, and with the final, 'Well, ladies and gentlemen, I think that concludes our business,' from the chairman, dispersing severally to other interrupted occupations. So, at a distance and in ignorance, might you vaguely picture the *Comité*'s work, hearing it casually mentioned. But of course your remoteness from the fact would be immense. Had this committee attempted to do all that is demanded of it by merely sitting round the table, its session would have been eternal, and its members long ago turned to stone.

Perhaps if we try to describe the routine of an ordinary day's work at No. 9 Knightsbridge, it will serve to suggest something of the range and compass of the committee's operations.

Let us suppose then that when, at a punctual nine o'clock in the morning, the purple-scarfed Boy Scout, who with so polite a firmness guards the door, lets in the arriving Director-General, we also, privileged with a discreet invisibility, are allowed to enter.

We are admitted to a narrow hall, of a business-like bareness, pervaded with the indefinable atmosphere of canvas bales and packing-cases, even when those very tangible objects do not obstruct your passage or meet you at full tilt, in hoisted above shirt-sleeves on muscular shoulders, as may happen at any moment.

We mount to the first floor. Facing us is the General Office: at our left is a door marked 'Inquiries.' We have many inquiries to make, but no one room will satisfy them; so we pass first into the front office, which with its three tall windows looks out on the trees of the Park. And here, seating ourselves beside the Director-General, and looking unabashed over his shoulder, we get a glimpse of his morning's correspondence. It is comprehensive and formidable.

But first there are some fifty '*Ordres de Mission*' to be signed.

What is an *Ordre de Mission*? It is a form which certifies that so-and-so, in the service of the Red Cross, is due to leave — and has to travel to —. The French railways, early in the war, made the valuable concession to the *Comité de Londres* and to the Anglo-French Committee, of allowing the workers sent out from England to travel free in France if armed with one of these vouchers. He or she presents the *Ordre de Mission* at the *Bureau Militaire* in the station of departure, and in return receives, after much filling in of coloured forms and many polite expressions, an Ordre de Transport which wafts the traveller, 'with horses and baggage' or 'without horses and baggage,' to his destination.

After dealing with these *Ordres de Mission*, the Director-General attacks his letters.

Many of these belong to the normal routine of one department or another, and are readily answered. Today, for instance, a firm writes that a new lorry has just been completed to order, and asks for a visit of inspection. A car is waiting at Le Havre for someone to fetch it: can that someone be sent over? Another is offered as a gift from Yorkshire, if that, too, can be fetched. A spare rim is wanted for a motor in the Marne district; tools and spare parts for another in the Midi. Timber is wanted by a unit at Salonika; a car of a certain type is wanted for purchase in London; estimates are submitted by one firm for an X-Ray car, by another for stoves, by yet another for various hospital equipment, and so on. Two drivers write to ask about their passports, their *fiches* and their *carnets*. The *fiche* is a paper of identification: but I dare not try to explain what the *carnet* is; it is just a little book that gives a great deal of trouble. There are gifts to be acknowledged, some from out-of-the-way parts of the world, and all corners of the Empire.

But there are also matters of more complexity, demanding careful thought and many-sided consideration. There are applications for work and offers of service. Men and women applying for specific posts, or now and again 'ready to go to France in any capacity.' It is a hard and unthankful thing to discourage goodwill, but goodwill alone is not, unfortunately, sufficient for 'any capacity.' Still, if a channel can be found for this offered energy, be sure it will be found.

Besides the units it controls, the *Comité* acts for groups and individuals doing special work; opens funds, keeps accounts, finds recruits. This involves much correspondence, of course, and there is correspondence too with committees and societies of kindred objects, and letters concerned with hospitals which have been taken over by the *Comité Britannique*, or which are being started by it.

These last matters, we surmise, are those most apt to furrow the Director-General's brow; but he has energy for all, and to spare. A long day's work is before him, and we leave him to attack it in detail.

At ten o'clock visitors begin to arrive at the office, and before long there may be five or six waiting in the anteroom. Their business is usually the business of getting out to France. In these days it is quite difficult enough to leave England at all, without the added difficulty of reaching a foreign destination. And to go out in a certain capacity under the Red Cross is to submit to an exhaustive scrutiny. We all know how necessary this sifting of credentials is. No good citizen will complain if the Red Cross is vigilant and scrupulous in selecting persons who are to be placed in a responsible position, and whose first duty it is to bear themselves discreetly; and the Anglo-French certificate is only granted, it need hardly be said, to those who can provide quite satisfactory proof of suitability. None the less, the normal Briton, accustomed to wander the world through without a question asked, takes but a gloomy satisfaction in precautions which, though they establish – superfluously, as he inclines to think – his good citizenship, make his journey out a sort of obstacle race. The *Comité*, however, saves the accepted applicant for service almost all his trouble. It is when the day for departure draws near that formalities suddenly thicken and complicate existence. The passport; the still more important visa for the passport; the certificate; the *fiche*; the *carnet*, mysterious and formidable; all these have to be procured and made out in proper order. Then the route; the uncertainty of the steamer's sailing up to the last moment – all the intricacies of correct travelling in war time; – these may well trouble and bewilder the novice going out for the first time. All hope is then centred on the Hon. Secretary, whom the waiters in the ante-room, patiently or impatiently, are now demanding to see and to be helped by. It is his department which sees to the various papers being made out in due form. It is he who resolves your uncertainties as to your features and complexion, when it comes to tabulations for passport purposes, and decides at a glance that your nose or your mouth is safely *'moyen.'* It is he who makes your way smooth at the Passport Office. Strange what a difference it makes which side of a door you are on! If we are in the ante-room, we share the impatience of those who have rashly counted on getting their business done in half an hour. How much more urgent surely is our mission than those of these others, who are being dealt with first, merely because they arrived before us! And how slow those officials are in the next room!

But in that next room we take quite another view, and we don't like being harassed with importunate messages, when work is to be got through which cannot be slurred and requires precision above all things.

It is someone's unthankful office to interview these visitors. Now and then there is one who bristles, who thinks it an indignity to be photographed, or who sees no need for references in the case of so manifest and proved a patriot; who has besides relations, so official, so important! And occasionally someone who has been working abroad brings a grievance, and is fluent with indignant speech. But these are exceptions on the whole singularly and surprisingly rare. And firm patience and sweet reason smooth all humours in time.

Another Honorary Secretary has under his eye the *dossier* of each of the hundreds of French hospitals which have applied for stores, clothing, etc., and deals with the correspondence relating to these matters, a correspondence which reaches ponderous dimensions. These applications come in daily, and are first submitted to *Madame la Présidente du Comité.*

If we descend for a moment to the ground floor, we shall find *Madame la Présidente* reigning in a room off the hall passage. It is her knowledge and judgment which guide the various departments – more than one, as we shall see – concerned in the hospital requisitions.

This work of supplying the needs of French hospitals is work that is also done by the French War Emergency Fund; but that fund does not concern itself with other than Military hospitals: any application it receives from a Red Cross hospital is at once sent on to the *Comité Britannique.*

The sifting of these requests is far from being the sole work with which *Madame la Présidente* charges herself. She holds all the threads of the *Comité's* activities. No one is so intimate with the condition of things in France; no one knows better the real needs of the sick and wounded; and with her large sympathy with the English people, her knowledge of the right persons to do the right things on both sides of the Channel, she has done and continues to do inestimable service to the cause of the friendship between the two nations. Without her help and direction it would have been impossible to guide and apply all the vast good-will and offered service of the British people to the destination where the needs of France are most urgent, in the way that the *Comité* has been able to do, without waste or friction. She has not only been the most devoted of workers but an inspiration to all she works with.

The requisition goes to *Madame la Présidente* first, who, if she approves of it, hands it to the *Pharmacie* and to one of the Hon. Secretaries to deal with clothing, to buy what is not in stock, and to give orders to the Packing Department, to pack ready for export the articles which are in stock.

Next we follow it upstairs to the second floor, to the *Pharmacie.* Such and such quantity of drugs is required for a hospital (say) in Central France. Here an order for the drugs is written out, when they are not in store; and when they are delivered, here they are packed. All war hospitals, of whatever kind, are supplied. In the year 1916, three hundred and forty-five Military hospitals were supplied with drugs, and four hundred and seventy-one hospitals belonging to the three Red Cross Societies.

On the wall of this room hangs a map of France. And into it are stuck flags denoting each a hospital to which drugs or clothes, or both, have been sent by the *Comité*; a small flag for a small hospital, a larger flag for a larger one. It is a tragic map. It opens a door on an horizon that appals. Who, with even the dullest imagination, could contemplate it, and see those little flags – thick as flowers in a June meadow, but of so desolate an import! – all over the departments of the country, and in places clustered in so close a swarm that the region mapped is altogether hidden; who could see these and think for a moment of what they mean – it is a nation silently bleeding in every member – and not feel a passionate sympathy with every effort to alleviate all that world of suffering?

It is not only drugs and dressings and invalid foods that are asked for and sent out. Here is a knock on the door that heralds a microscope, ready packed in its box, which will shortly be doing good service for the Carrel treatment of wounds, in a sector of the front. Microscopes are today very difficult to get; all the more will this one be prized. Sometimes a whole X-Ray outfit will be sent out. And besides directly medical aid, games, books, note-paper, are packed and despatched. These things are immensely appreciated at the actual front. A lieutenant or an *aumônier* gets to know that they may be procured for the men through this channel. He writes to the *Comité*, and his request, whether for a football or for picture postcards, is immediately answered. The '*Paquetage du Soldat*,' at 5 Princes Gate, is the *Comité*'s branch for this work – financed by the *Comité* and domiciled in the *Présidente*'s house.

It is in this room, for lack of space, that the Matron, on three days in the week, interviews every nurse going out.

Next door, and on every floor, are the typists, always busy. And upstairs are two departments; concerned, one with the Accountant, and the other with purchase of stores. But now we must resume the fortunes of the requisition sheet which arrived this morning. The list of drugs demanded has been made out. But there is also a demand for clothes; and clothes are the care of a separate department. We descend therefore to the basement, where we find the lady in charge busy in a room lined with cupboards. The cupboards are full of 'clothing' – a liberal term, including blankets, sheets, pillows, towels, napkins, as well as lengths of flannel, calico, and other material. Much of this is bought, much given. We see in one of the cupboards great heaps of shirts and pyjamas, sent as a gift from Australia. These are woollen and of admirable quality.

Each type of 'clothing' is done up in bundles of tens, for convenience and rapidity of packing. In this work there are ladies who volunteer their help. It is a work which is always urgent, for the house contains so little room for storage that arriving parcels have to be handled with the least possible delay.

Each set of goods requisitioned by a hospital is sorted out and got ready, and then sewn up in canvas. We pass to a small room at the back – flattening ourselves against the wall as a boy hurries past with a voluminous load of pillows sticking out in all directions – and there we find the packers at work. On an average fifty bales a day are packed; and, with those that come ready packed, over 1000 packages a week are sent to France from 9 Knightsbridge.

Mounting again, we find the hall full of bales and cases. Some of these have come addressed to some particular hospital in France, and are merely forwarded by the committee. But then there are many cases of mixed goods, which are sent in by various hospital supply depots; these have to be unpacked, sorted, and stored in the various departments, to await a speedy despatch. It is the task of one of the staff to superintend the sorting and addressing of the bales.

Insinuating ourselves into the General Office once more, we find the Director-General interviewing a surgeon who has returned on leave, and who has some difficulty with the mesh of formalities apt to entangle the unwary traveller. He is in the process of being extricated and made happy.

One of the Hon. Secretaries is reassuring a prospective orderly. But another department, hitherto unvisited, claims our attention.

The *Comité* has sent over 500 motor cars of various types to France. Each car has its *dossier* here; and there is a card index, with a triple entry; under the maker of the car, the person who took it out, and the unit to which it is attached. This, of course, must be kept up to date.

The three members of the staff, who divide the cares of this department, test the efficiency of prospective drivers and make all the arrangements for the passage of the car to France. And perhaps this is as good an opportunity as any to say something of a branch of the manifold activities of the *Comité* which might easily escape attention. This is work done by cars with English drivers who are not attached to the convoys working with the French armies on the Western Front and in the Balkans, or to any of the Anglo-French hospitals.

In almost every department of France, the *Comité* has ambulances or touring cars working, some under their local *délégué*, others attached to Red Cross or Military *Formations Sanitaires*. The drivers are all volunteers, and many give their own cars. They convey wounded to and from stations, and doctors to remote hospitals, and they do all sorts of transport work, as, for example, in the XVIth and XVIIth *Régions*. Perpignan, Albi, Castres, Mende, Montpellier, are some of the centres served. The region is mostly mountainous. At Prades, patients suffering from eczema and other skin diseases are taken up to baths in the mountains, ten kilometres away, and brought back again in relays. One car does three journeys in the day. At Rodez there is a small English staff and a well-equipped operating theatre. At Montpellier two English workers are engaged on what the French call *mécano-thérapie*. At Palavas, on the Mediterranean coast, there is a large hospital devoted to tuberculous cases, with a terrace for sun-baths facing full south; and here a great part of the nursing staff is English. Besides the cars attached to the several centres, a perfectly-equipped X-Ray car has recently been sent out for the service of those hospitals which need it. This car makes a circuit of the region.

At Marseilles, again, an English lady is doing devoted service, keeping her own car in order, and working ten hours a day.

It is needless to add that such extensions of the *Comité*'s activities – and these examples could be multiplied almost indefinitely – in addition to all the work of the convoys and the cars attached to hospitals, mean a vast amount of correspondence.

Now that all these departments are in full tide of work, we will take the opportunity of slipping out to No. 3, a few doors off, where three departments accessory to the work of the *Comité* are lodged.

One of these is concerned with Prisoners of War. We all know what a boon and support, what an actual necessity very often are the parcels of food, tobacco, etc., sent out by their friends to prisoners in the enemy countries. Since March 1917, control of the despatch from England of all such parcels to French prisoners of war has been officially handed over to the *Comité Britannique*.

Naturally this department is mainly concerned with prisoners who before the war were domiciled in England, or who have friends and relations in this country. Such friends and relations have the choice of either buying, at the cost of five shillings, one of the standard parcels of food supplied by the French Red Cross, or of obtaining from the department a permit to buy the particular articles they want to send from one of the shops officially authorised to pack parcels for prisoners. The amount of food is limited to sixty pounds in every four weeks. Not more than 8 ounces of tobacco, and not more than 300 cigarettes, may be sent each fortnight.

But this department of the *Comité* does more than act as an official channel for gifts: it gives itself. And nothing, I think, is more expressive of the animating spirit of the

Comité than this spontaneous seeking out of the means to help those unhappy men in the German prison camps. Many of the French prisoners come from the invaded regions; their homes are deserted, or shattered to dust and fragments; their wives and children are refugees; and the bitterest of their lot is to know that those who would naturally be the helpers and comforters of their sufferings are more helpless and comfortless than themselves. It is these especially, with any others who have no friends or kinsfolk to help them, whom this department tries to find, and to whom it sends free parcels. Among the friendless ones are many soldiers of the native African regiments of the French army. They get to know from comrades of this means of aid, and write to the *Comité*, asking for a parcel. Here is one who writes, half in English, half in French: 'Please, I am come from *Algeries*. My country is very far from here.' I am glad to know that a parcel is on its way to that poor Algerian in his German prison.

With each parcel is sent a postcard, so that the prisoners may acknowledge the receipt of it. They are asked to state if the parcels come regularly and in good condition. Earlier in the year (1917) the replies were occasionally disappointing. One wrote: '*Le contenu était en bon état – confisqué par les autorités.*' And another: ' *En bon état. Les Allemands ont tout gardé. Ils appellent cela représailles. On m'a laissé la boîte d'emballage.*' But recently conditions seem greatly to have bettered. Very few of the postcards now contain complaints. And the warm words of gratitude that come daily from the prisoners testify to the good work done.

In each of the camps there is a Prisoners' Committee, and the department is in touch with the presidents of these committees, so as to ensure that free parcels are not being sent to any who are already sufficiently supplied with food from friends in France.

And what does this work amount to? Well, we find that each week the department is sending out about six hundred parcels, of a total value of £150. Two hundred of these are paid for by friends, four hundred are sent free by the *Comité*. Then there are the parcels sent out, as already explained, by friends and relatives under the permit system. These represent a monthly value of £125. And besides the food, there are also parcels of clothing sent out – especially warm underclothing and boots, at the rate of about a hundred a month.

We have now to see the department which deals with the canteens. Much of this work is new; fresh canteens are always being started, and old canteens are continually being moved from place to place under orders from the French authorities. This all involves many letters and telegrams. But the main business of the gentleman who has this department in his charge is to find 'Canteeners,' to interview ladies who contemplate going out, to arrange where they are to go, how they are to reach their destination, and how the work is to be organised when they have arrived. We shall have much more to say of the canteens later on.

The office of the canteens is on the ground floor of No. 3; and the two upper floors are devoted to the *ouvroir*. In these workrooms a number of ladies, most of them members of the French colony in London, make clothing and bandages for the wounded. Similar work is being done at branch offices, and great quantities of such necessaries are always being sent out to the French hospitals, the fruit of these patient labours.

And now we pass to another office at 34 Wilton Place, where we find a department devoted to France's Day.

You will be surprised perhaps that the celebration of the Fourteenth of July in Britain, with its collections for the French Red Cross, should keep a permanent staff engaged throughout the year. But so it is. And when you have heard a few details of what it all entails, you will not wonder any more. For one thing, though the Day is celebrated in London on the fourteenth of July, the celebrations in the provinces are held on various dates, even as late, this last year, in the case of at least one town, as 15th December. Then the preparations are on an enormous scale. There are millions of trays and souvenirs to be manufactured, packed and sent out. The Mayors of the provincial cities and towns must be applied to; centres must be created, with depots in each centre, and an organised subdivision of the work in districts: an infinity of correspondence! The department has a depot in St. James's Street, where the packing is done: and the packing occupies three or four months. Few people have any notion of what the word 'million' really means, even in these days when it comes to our lips so glibly. A few thousands, actually realised 'in the flesh,' so to speak, are quite enough for our minds to deal with; and when it comes to nine million penny souvenirs, the two or three million of threepenny, the million of sixpenny, the two million of more expensive specimens, it is 'a thing imagination boggles at.' We can only marvel, and admire the patience and the enterprise of the devoted worker, who arranges these immensities. Even so, we have omitted the masses of bills and posters, which are no mean item of the business. It is pleasant to learn that all parts of England have vied with each other in generosity for the sake of the wounded of France.

On the 15th of October last, there was a little gathering at the French Embassy, where Monsieur Cambon, in his own quiet, cordial, gracious way, acknowledged on behalf of his country the gifts of the British people. After enumerating some of the chief contributions and describing the range and scope of the work done, he continued:

> 'More than two thousand people are employed by the London Committee of the *Croix Rouge Française* in France and in England. They carry out every kind of work in a spirit of absolute disinterestedness, so that we cannot thank them otherwise than by telling them how deeply grateful we are for their help. We cannot do more here. At the headquarters of the committee, close by here, in Knightsbridge, more than eighty people are devoting their time to the service of the *Croix Rouge*. It is a great organisation. I will not name any one because I would have to name everybody, and they are all very retiring and disinterested people, who would feel embarrassed by the expression of my thanks....
>
> 'Everybody works with truly wonderful dash and enthusiasm. French and English ladies work side by side, learning to appreciate one another, working in a true spirit of fraternity. The spectacle of all this devotion, this disinterestedness, truly inspires one with a deep regard for human nature. There are pessimists, you know, who will always abuse human nature. I think they are mistaken. As soon as there are misfortunes to relieve, men and women alike realise their duty, and every form of selfishness disappears....'

In the first year of the war, when the business of organising 'France's Day' had not yet been handed over to the *Comité de Londres*, the net amount collected was £24,115. In 1916 it was £104,111. In 1917 it was £190,349. 1918 is to do still better!

BRITISH NURSES IN FRANCE

THE FRENCH FLAG NURSING CORPS

Before describing the growth of the convoys and hospitals it will be well to give some account of an important society or association formed after the outbreak of war, which has aimed at helping France not by fitting out separate units, controlled from Britain, but by placing workers at the disposal of the French authorities.

The French Flag Nursing Corps owes its origin to an Englishwoman, who was educated in France, and who is known to many as the author of a book on her experiences of Turkish life. This lady, with whom the writer had a talk in Paris, told him of the things she had seen in France during the battles of the Marne; of the journey to Bordeaux – a fifty-five hours' journey – on a train which had no food on board, and of the severely wounded men to whose hurts there had been no time to attend.

In the first days of the war, the lady who is well known as the President of the National Council of Trained Nurses of Great Britain and Ireland, foreseeing the likelihood of the need, had offered thoroughly trained English nurses to various authorities in France; but at that moment it was supposed that existing arrangements would suffice, and these offers were declined. The event overwhelmed all anticipations. During the great retreat, and the battles of the Marne, the Red Cross, like the transport service, and the municipal authorities everywhere, was put to a fearful strain.

Without the well-appointed hospital trains which the

needs of the war have since created; without motor ambulances – carried in jolting carts, or lying in the straw of cattle-trucks, the lot of the wounded in those days hardly bears to be imagined.

Here is a little glimpse of what was happening, day and night – a glimpse of suffering that was but an infinitesimal fraction of the whole. It is a correspondent of the *Daily Telegraph* who writes, and who describes what he saw at a station fifteen miles from Paris. He was helping French and American women to give food and drink to the wounded:

> Towards the end of the train were carriages where no faces appeared at the windows, and on opening the doors one saw some ragged and helpless victim of the war lying amid straw, crying feebly for drink, and asking if there at last was the hospital where his sufferings were to end.
>
> Farther back still were the great cattle wagons which, when opened, revealed six, eight, or even more men lying helpless in the straw, sometimes in total darkness, sometimes lighted by one lantern, the pale rays of which only added to the horrors of the scene! How can I describe the condition of these men?
>
> In one wagon eight of them were uniting in a chorus of suffering. We could hear them before we had slid back the great wooden doors, like voices crying from the tomb.... For nearly two days they had been in this dark and airless cattle-wagon, burned by fever, their wounds throbbing and stabbing with every movement of the train.... One man had relieved himself of all clothing in the intensity of his fever, and was tossing about naked in the straw. I wrapped

him up in a blanket and gave him some hot milk....

All through the night train after train rolled in from the battlefield. By seven in the morning, when others relieved us, thirteen trains, containing over three thousand wounded, had passed. Three thousand at one station in a single night. So it has been going on day and night for over fourteen days, and these are only the victims of one section of the battlefield.

The most perfect organisation cannot prevent such tortures; it can only mitigate them. And for the moment the means of destruction had far exceeded the means of mitigation.

If an unparalleled strain was put on the transport service, the hospitals – mostly improvised – which received the wounded were not less hardly driven.

There was unlimited devotion, immense eagerness to serve; but of trained and expert help there was an inevitable deficiency. The ladies of Paris staffed the Red Cross hospitals, and did all they could. It was the same in other towns. Some of the most devoted nursing work in those days was done, let it be recorded, by women of the streets. But the crying need was for skill, training, experience. And it is told how a Frenchwoman, who knew what nursing requirements really were, and who had seen a well-appointed English ambulance train, sat and wept because so many of her dear countrymen lacked the comforts and the help they so sorely needed.

It was this condition of things which inspired the English lady of whom we have already spoken with the idea of the French Flag Nursing Corps. She went to the head of the French Army Medical Corps, and proposed to procure for the French wounded a large number of fully trained British nurses, to work in French military hospitals for the duration of the war. The offer was eagerly accepted. Work began in October 1914. Seven nurses, under the direction of a sister, went to Rouen, and gave much valued assistance to the nuns who were nursing in that district. A few months after, one of the largest hospitals in the Gironde region was placed at the disposal of the English nurses by the Ministry of War.

It was an opportunity for testing the value of skilled nursing in war time: and the testimony of the French doctors and surgeons, under whom they have worked, shows what precious metal the test revealed. On their side, the sisters profited by the chance of becoming acquainted with French methods, as practised by distinguished surgeons.

Nurses of the Corps were now beginning to go out to France in a steady stream; and to cope with the growth of the work, the sister who had been in command at Rouen was appointed Matron-in-Chief of the Corps.

In temporary French hospitals along the firing line, as well as at many towns in the interior, these nurses are to be found. They have to contend with daily difficulties, over and above their hard service; difficulties which in the early months of the war were aggravated tenfold by circumstances.

Picture the English nurse as we know her, trained to an exacting standard, accomplished in every detail of her profession, and accustomed to have at her hand all necessary material and appliances, and to follow a settled routine. Picture her plunged into a foreign land, among strangers whose tongue she perhaps understands and speaks but imperfectly – you may see her snatching a few minutes of scarce rest to improve her French with grammar and phrase-book; picture her in a hospital improvised for the war, installed in a building designed for quite other uses, full of makeshift devices, inadequately clean, too probably, from disuse; picture her confronted with a desperate pressure of work, severe cases coming in every day, and confronted besides with all the difficulties of unaccustomed methods, and under strange direction. You can imagine that this was no light undertaking.

A difference of race, a difference of temperament like that which exists between the French and English, takes time to understand and allow for. Differences of custom and of religion also provide subtle opportunities for bruised feeling. There was also the prejudice against professional nursing, which has been already mentioned, and which had to be overcome.

To run an improvised war hospital is not so difficult for a trained sister when she has the control of it; but to work in such a hospital without independence is a very different matter. Add to all this the fact that in the first few weeks of the war the best-equipped hospitals, with all their store of chloroform, gauze, and surgical appliances, had been taken by the Germans in their invading march; and the enemy's possession of the chief manufacturing districts made it hard to replenish those stores with any sufficiency.

Our dear imperfect human nature betrays its weaknesses in such a situation, but how much more does it show the good undaunted stuff of which it is made!

If at first there was a tendency to regard British methods as superfluously scrupulous and thorough – and so perversely are we compounded that we do not always enjoy being done good to, especially if old habits are invaded; if there were differences of theory as to the value of fresh air; and if English nurses, on their part, made sometimes too little allowance for conditions of war, and expected too near a conformity with their accustomed standards; this is no cause for wonder. Even war breaks custom hardly. But what may well cause wonder is that, with so many occasions of difficulty, things came to run so smoothly as on the whole they have done. The Sisters won their way to confidence by the excellence of their work. 'Their well-directed energy, their self-sacrifice have never wavered,' wrote a French doctor, and his testimony is but one of many. A high official wrote: 'The nurses of the French Flag Nursing Corps are considered by the doctors of our armies as assistants of the first class, and their presence in France, in a number the insufficiency of which we regret, is one of the most touching evidences of the sympathy of the English nation towards our country.'

Of particular value was the work done by those nurses in fever hospitals; for in fever cases the nurse counts for even more than the doctor; and here the trained skill of the English nurse saved many a life.

Since the nurses of this Corps are scattered among so many different French units, it is impossible to write a history of their work, though with a little imagination one can picture what it has been, and what it has meant. But we must not omit to mention the two hospital barges which were staffed by nurses of the Corps, and which transported the seriously wounded along the canal from Adinkerke to Bourbourg; nor the hospitals at Bergues, where the nurses carried down the wounded into the cellars under the fire of the German bombardment – hospitals which the Sisters had so splendidly transformed, and which unhappily, owing to the bombardments, had to be closed and abandoned.

Early in 1917 the French Flag Nursing Corps was taken over from its old committee by the *Comité de Londres*. The nurses' salaries are now paid by the *Comité* instead of, as formerly, by the French Government.

This may be the fittest place to remind the reader that, besides all this skilled service by the trained nurses of the French Flag Nursing Corps, a great amount of work has been done in French hospitals by English people who have given their personal services, not only as nurses, but in a dozen different capacities. These have been people who had their homes in France, and attached themselves to some hospital in their own neighbourhood, doing whatever seemed most needful in that particular place; or else they happened to be staying in some particular district when war broke out, or knew of a hospital which needed help.

PART II

THE RECORD

THE CONVOYS

THE FIRST YEAR

It became known in England in the early months of the war that more ambulances for the wounded were urgently required for the French Army's unprecedented needs.

The Automobile Association learning of this want in October 1914, appealed at once to their members to provide touring cars which might be converted into ambulance cars. About two hundred and fifty cars were offered to the committee: and a very large number of members, who could not provide cars, subscribed between them over six thousand pounds. Some small proportion of the cars offered were rejected, as it was difficult to convert them; but over two hundred were in the end shipped to France. The Association's engineering department collected the cars by road and rail from all parts of the country, converted them into ambulances, overhauled and equipped them.

The first fifty cars were inspected by the King in the grounds of Buckingham Palace. As they were completed, the cars were driven to Southampton, shipped thence to Havre, and there handed over to the *Service de Santé*. At that point unfortunately they disappear from our view, to run who knows what thousands of miles, carrying their freight of wounded.

In the case of the convoys, whose story we have now to tell, we are able to follow the ambulances and know what work they did, because they were not merely handed over to the French, but were driven by Englishmen. Particular mention must here be made of the British Ambulance

Committee, an independent body formed expressly to provide convoys for French wounded, not behind the lines but on the actual front. It owes its existence to its present Inspector-General, who in September 1917 went to Bordeaux and made proposals to the military authorities. It was a hard thing to procure permission for civilians to serve in the conditions desired; it was against all precedent; but persuasive perseverance won in the end. The influential Committee formed, with headquarters at 23A Bruton Street, has obtained splendid support from its friends and the public, amounting to more than £300,000. The first complete British convoys attached to the French Army on the model of its own *Sections Sanitaires* were those of this Committee. Its five convoys were sent out in the first half of 1915, and were numbered 1 to 5 of the *Sections Sanitaires Anglaises*, their fine work being immediately recognised. During 1915, other British volunteer convoys which had sought and found work with the French in the first months of the war, on a less official basis, were brought into the system thus inaugurated. The units were re-grouped and organised in sections, as we shall see. In order to tell things in their sequence, we shall begin with these pioneer enterprises.

It must be added that most liberal help in the provision of ambulance cars has come from the fund known as the Dennis Bayley Fund, now a branch of the British Red Cross Society and Order of St. John. Through the energy of the founder of this fund, and of his lieutenant, great industrial firms – both owners and workers – were canvassed throughout England, and asked to make a voluntary levy on output or wages to support the cause of the transport of the wounded. The great industries of Britain have magnificently responded to this invitation. Over half a million pounds has been raised almost entirely by these industries, headed by the coal-owners of Nottinghamshire and Derbyshire; and this sum has been devoted to providing convoys for the British, French, and Italian fronts. Of the convoys supplied for working with the French, four and a half have been given to the British Red Cross Society, one convoy and a motor-cycle section to the British Ambulance Committee. These convoys are all maintained by the fund, and it is also undertaking the maintenance of the convoy known as Section 10, which was organised by the British Committee of the French Red Cross. We shall see what severe work the convoys have to do, and what invaluable support this fund has given. The members of Lloyd's also gave two convoys to the British Ambulance Committee; and the British Farmers' Red Cross Fund gave another to the British Committee of the French Red Cross.

In the quite early days of the war, in those pregnant and breathless weeks which followed the battle of the Marne, ambulances of the British Red Cross were already assisting the French field hospitals in certain districts.

In September 1914 a detachment was appointed by the British Red Cross Society to undertake the work of searching for missing and wounded, and also to register graves of the dead, from Ghent to Amiens. Towards the end of the month, the Commandant, being at Amiens, was asked by the French to assist them in evacuating their wounded from Albert. That town had been suddenly attacked with great force by the Germans.

The moment was one of the most critical in the war. It was the moment when the Allied armies had begun their wide outflanking movement to the West and North. The frontal assault on those strong positions to which the Germans had fallen back, on the heights beyond the Aisne, had, as we all know, quickly subsided into the sullen stationary warfare of the trenches. About the middle of September, the French command resolved on a new stroke. The line was lengthened on the left, fresh forces were brought up; from Compiégne northward, through Roye and Albert, the extended armies threatened the outflanked German right. On the 30th of September, and for some days following, furious battles disputed the possession of the Albert plateau.

Such was the situation when the aforesaid unit was asked to help the French at Albert with their wounded. It was at once decided to form a mobile hospital attached to the unit. This mobile hospital changed its headquarters from time to time. During most of October it was at Hesdin, and from there helped the French field hospitals east of Doullens, as well as in the Arras region, and in places still farther north. The mobile unit used, at its fullest working, sixteen motor ambulances and four staff cars. The way it worked was this: Officers in charge of the ambulances reported to the French officers at their several field hospitals and aidposts, and took their orders. The wounded were then transported to the appointed hospitals and evacuation points. Drivers and orderlies helped in the stretcher-work. Severe cases were brought to the mobile hospital and treated by British doctors. All this was being done close behind the front, with continuous hard fighting going on; so it may be imagined that the pressure was severe, and patients were evacuated as soon as they were fit to be moved, to make room for the urgent cases incessantly coming in.

The devoted work of the unit was warmly appreciated,

not only for the 'swiftness and comfort' with which the wounded were carried, but for the 'spontaneity and warmth' of the English offers of aid. A French army doctor wrote to thank the unit's commander for the 'precious help' it had given. The British ambulances had transported more than one hundred and fifty wounded to Amiens and to Doullens in three days. 'By this action,' the doctor wrote, 'you have greatly relieved our own convoys and secured a very swift and continuous evacuation for the severely wounded, some of whom, I do not scruple to say, will owe their recovery to you.' He went on to thank the English doctors for placing their services at the disposal of their French *confrères*, and enabling the overtaxed French medical staff to snatch a few hours' rest.

The mobile unit continued to work for the French during the autumn of 1914, and the spring of the following year. During part of the time it also evacuated a number of British wounded. It may be remembered that the strategic movements leading up to, and following, the battle of the Marne, had resulted in the British Army being, at the end of September, no longer on the extreme left of the French line, but almost at its centre. Early in October it was transferred, by a brilliantly smooth operation, to its old place on the extreme left; and the crossing of French and English lines of communication no longer made confusion in the rear. The Ypres salient, however, was for a certain period, from mid-November to the end of January, held by French troops.

On the 3rd of March 1915 a section of five motor ambulances went south to Chalons, and worked there till the 6th of May, carrying French wounded to and from various points. But the mobile unit ceased working for the French armies in March, and in May it was disbanded.

Meanwhile the race to the coast – the result of the French outflanking movement and the answering movement of the Germans – had been won – how narrowly! – by the Allies; Antwerp had fallen; the First Battle of Ypres, in which the British Army, attacked by forces at least four times as numerous, so magnificently held firm the line to the sea, had overthrown the German's second plan of campaign as decisively as the Marne had overthrown their first.

One of the most moving and magnificent episodes of the battles for the coast was, as everyone knows, the defence of Dixmude by the French *Fusiliers Marins*. With that famous defence, and with that valiant corps certain Britons are proud to have been associated. The French Naval Brigade, commanded by Admiral Ronarc'h, arrived in Ghent to reinforce the Belgians, on 8th October. In that town an English volunteer unit, known as the Munro Ambulance Corps, had been already for some weeks at work, busily engaged in bringing in the wounded from the villages in the neighbourhood, which day by day were falling into the enemy's hands. Antwerp was burning, and the Germans were advancing westward, while the Allies – Belgian, French and British – slowly retreated. The Fusiliers took up a position at Melle, a little town close to, and in front of, Ghent. There, in a spirited action they not only barred the German advance, but even drove the enemy back a few miles, and by this resistance gave the retiring Belgian army forty-eight hours' start.

The young Breton sailors, now proving their mettle under fire for the first time, had been made into an infantry brigade on an emergency; they had been re-equipped as soldiers in haste; and they had no ambulances for their wounded. The Commandant (and founder) of the Munro Ambulance Corps therefore offered its services to the Fusiliers; and thus began an association which lasted through many months of strenuous warfare.

The fight at Melle saved valuable time, but there was no question of attempting to stand on these positions. Legions of Germans were coming up on both banks of the Scheldt, and only retreat could save the Allied forces from being cut off. The Fusiliers, for the moment under the command of an English General, retired through Ghent, an English division covering their retreat and following them at an interval of two hours.

The members of the Munro Corps shared the trials of this retreat in the autumn rain, driving their cars along congested roads, where stupefied peasants, with their earthly goods in bundles on their backs, fleeing from their homes they knew not whither, and conscious only of the terrible enemy behind, kept themselves moving alongside the marching troops. More than once it was intended to stand and fight; but the Germans were advancing in overwhelming force; and no satisfactory line of defence was found till the Yser was reached. The line ran from Nieuport through Dixmude to Ypres. At Furnes, the little old town of fine architecture, which before the war was famed for its sacred pageant and procession in July – a relic of the Middle Ages – the Munro Corps found its new headquarters. Furnes is at about an equal distance from Nieuport and from Dixmude. Through the battle of the Yser and the First Battle of Ypres, the Corps, which at this time numbered about twenty cars, worked day and night for French, English, and Belgians. A great number of ambulances had been abandoned during the retreat, and the lack of them was bitterly felt during those weeks of desperate effort and incessant fighting. The cars of the Corps, half of which were lent by the British Red Cross Society, did precious service for the wounded, whose sufferings and discomforts – as a member of the Corps, who was from August 1915 its Commandant, has recorded – were quite indescribable. Much of the general work from Furnes was irregular and contingent on the needs of the moment, but a regular evacuation service was maintained for the French military hospitals in the town. The Corps devoted itself more especially to the aid of the *Fusiliers Marins* during their epical defence of Dixmude, from 16th October to 10th November, when six thousand French sailors and a lesser number of Belgian soldiers, without any heavy guns, without aeroplanes, in fabulous morasses of mud, under never-ending rain, held up three entire Army Corps of Germans fighting their hardest to break through, at this most vulnerable point, to Dunkirk and Calais. Dixmude fell, battered to pieces; but the superb endurance of the garrison had won its object.

In December, first a battalion, then the entire brigade, of *Fusiliers Marins* was sent to Nieuport. They still had no regimental ambulances; and Admiral Ronarc'h asked the Munro Corps to undertake once more the evacuation of the wounded from the dressing stations to the clearing hospitals. At first this service was carried on by a few cars only, but later other cars were added, according to need.

At Nieuport the Corps continued to work through 1915 till November, when the Naval Brigade was reduced to a battalion. The Corps was asked to continue its work for the troops which relieved the Brigade. It had worked with the *Fusiliers Marins* under a simple agreement or understanding; but it was now necessary that matters should be placed on a more regular and official footing. One section of six cars passed under the entire control of the French, and was placed in a barrack within three miles of the front. There it evacuated wounded from the dressing stations in Nieuport to the clearing hospitals.

There was another small English convoy which did fine service during the tremendous days of that autumn. This was the Millicent Sutherland Ambulance, whose earlier adventures in Belgium will be found recorded in our story of the hospitals. The convoy of four ambulances and a large omnibus for sitting cases (afterwards increased to eight cars) was taken out by the lady who founded and who still directs the unit, and landed at Dunkirk on 23rd October. The cars ran day and night from field hospitals near the Yser front, bringing back wounded to Dunkirk and Zuydecote, and to the hospital ships, which then sailed to Cherbourg. Endless trains of cattle-trucks filled with the wounded were then arriving at Dunkirk station, where the directress of this unit and her helpers started canteen work for those most pitiable sufferers. The convoy afterwards did good work at Malo, near Dunkirk, till late in 1915, when the unit transferred its services to the British.

But we must now return to the activities of the British Red Cross Unit. The original second in command of that first detachment took control of a unit of motor ambulances which was attached, early in October 1914, to the *Service de Santé* of the Second Army. The unit contained a certain number of American volunteers.

For the first few months after being attached to the Second Army – that is, during the autumn and early winter of 1914 – this unit was busy evacuating wounded from field hospitals to Compiègne, Montdidier, Amiens, and

Doullens. From Compiègne in the south to Doullens in the north is roughly sixty miles, Amiens and Montdidier lying at almost equidistant points between the two, but a little farther from the front. Doullens was made the headquarters, but a sub-division of cars was stationed at Montdidier. The gigantic German effort to break through to the coast spent itself during the second half of November. For the rest of the year the fighting was on a smaller scale. With the coming of the cold weather trenches were deepened and elaborated, on both sides, with all the devices of the skilled engineer. But the enemy was never left idle; there was incessant sniping, with a big toll of dead and wounded; the guns continued their unending duel; and there was plenty of work for the ambulances to do. During the last days of December the pressure became heavy; more than once one of the convoys was working for twenty-four hours on end. The French General wrote to the Commandant his appreciation of the unit's services.

In May Doullens was taken into the zone of another army. The unit was ordered to move, but found little doing at its new headquarters. The serious fighting was north of Arras, where, beginning on the 9th, a brilliant French offensive thrust at Lens, and made the bloodiest of fighting about Souchez, and Carency, and Notre Dame de Lorette.

The call for ambulances was urgent, and a request for help came to the unit from the Doullens district. With the consent of the Second Army Command, the ambulances were sent to help this other part of the line, and came in for heavy and continuous work both by night and day.

Late in May the unit was again moved. According to the orders of the General in command, a number of ambulances were now stationed at certain posts close to the trenches.

Each of these dealt with such casualties as occurred in the neighbourhood of its post. They were relieved every twenty-four hours. The rest of the convoy, posted some five kilometres back, was held in readiness for a summons coming from any part of the line served.

During June the strength of the unit was greatly increased. At the beginning of the month it had eighteen ambulances, four touring cars, a motor lorry, and a motor kitchen-car. By the end of the month these twenty-four cars had been increased to thirty-three.

In mid-September the unit was found new quarters at Somme Vesle (having moved several times during the summer); and its strength was further increased to fifty-three ambulances and five touring cars. The work was now carried on among villages wrecked and devastated since the first weeks of the war. Accommodation for the staff was difficult to find among the shattered cottages and roofless barns. It became necessary to buy tents. The conditions were trying, the work heavy. But the French Command had taken note of the work and the workers; and on September 20th the Commandant was told that it had been decided to make his unit responsible for the service of a whole Army Corps, instead of sharing it, as hitherto, with a French section.

A few days later the unit was moved to Champagne.

It was the eve of the great Champagne attack which opened on the morning of 25th September, coinciding with the British attack at Loos in the north. The attack was timed for 8a.m.; and by nine in the evening, all the ambulances were at their required stations. Fifteen ambulances were distributed among four field hospitals, and fourteen more were equally divided between two posts at certain communication trenches. It was important to find cover from aircraft for the ambulances when they were parked together: at the same time the camps had to be close to the track followed by the cars between communication trench and field hospital, and not near a battery, in case of its drawing concentrated shell-fire. These conditions were not easy to satisfy.

La Champagne Pouilleuse, that singular region of Eastern France which retains among the fertile lands surrounding it something primevally forlorn, is a country of bare rolling hills and shallow valleys, patched with meagre fir plantations. Such villages as there were had been obliterated in the war. The patches of fir were useful for screening the ambulances from aerial observation. But the batteries assembled for the great attack were posted so closely together that it was impossible to station the cars far from any one of them. Bomb-proof shelters were, however, provided. And, as it turned out, the reply of the German guns to the French artillery was surprisingly ineffective.

A system of new roads – for of old ones there were hardly any – as well as of light railways, had been constructed along the front. The chalky, powdery soil, turned into slippery mud by the least rain, is in fine weather remarkably dusty. And this September the weather had been continuously fine, with bright sun and cool nights for some weeks. But on the evening of the 24th, when the ambulances took their appointed positions, heavy rain began to fall. The wind had changed to the south-west. Every unit now had its orders. The roads were thronged with an endless movement of ammunition trains, of revictualling convoys, of columns of infantry and squadrons of cavalry. The guns along the whole line kept up a continuous cannonade.

Darkness fell. A little after midnight the bombardment increased to a terrible intensity. From the masses of troops behind the front, regiments began to move up along the communication trenches. With the break of day it became possible to distinguish the German lines stretching along the ridge of the opposite downs.

It was a dripping cheerless morning, and the powdery chalk, now churned into heavy slime, was slippery going for the feet. But when the artillery ceased, to lengthen range, and in the sudden astonishing silence the lines of French infantry – along a front of fifteen miles – sprang out of the trenches and went forward, it was with a confidence and momentum that made them irresistible.

A little way back, beside the communication trenches, the English ambulances, now promoted to serve a whole Army Corps, were waiting. It was not long before the wounded began to arrive. The French had taken the enemy first-line trenches at a blow; but machine-guns and shells from the big guns in the rear had grievously thinned the ranks of their advance. Three ambulances were kept always waiting at each communication trench; as soon as one was filled and left, another came up from the camping ground and took its place. But before this first day of the battle was over, the seven cars assigned to each communication trench proved quite insufficient. At one post the number was increased to ten, at another to twelve.

With the wounded came also prisoners, unnerved and stupefied by the bombardment and by hunger; for the French guns had cut off their supplies for some days. The Commandant reported that 'amongst the prisoners taken was the complete staff equipment of a German Field Hospital,' and among the trophies were devices for protection from gas and for administering treatment to those suffering from its effects. And specially to be noted is this. One of the portable 'gas-projectors' bore the date 1915. But an inscription on it recorded that the pattern of this date superseded the pattern of 1912, which in its turn superseded that of 1910. Long ago, in days of peace, the Germans were brewing their poison-gas.

Imagine now the work before our men, on this day of fine rain which soaked into the white sticky soil, as the stream of wounded, some carried on stretchers, others stumbling along with bandaged head or arm, thickened and grew to a steady volume. All day they were arriving, and on through the night; and the next day and the next night; and still there was no rest for the drivers of the cars. Only after five days and five nights was the pressure relaxed. By then, the great attack had spent its force; and though the last lines of the enemy had been actually breached at one point, the breach was not wide enough, and the Germans soon had it blocked by their reserves. During these five days the British convoy with its wounded covered more than thirty thousand kilometres. They worked day and night on roads which, even before the first wounded had begun to come in, had been so broken up by the incessant heavy traffic and the pouring rain that they were poached into deep holes full of water. The traffic never ceased; the roads were densely packed with moving cars and wagons; the mud grew deeper and more slippery; no lights were allowed by night. In such conditions our Red Cross men steered their cars and drove their wounded night and day. Those who worked at the two communication trenches were unable to take off their clothes for nine days. For the battle still went on, after the manner of the battles of this war, which have no definite end, but smoulder down into the stationary warfare from which they began. But the casualties were now lighter. On the 8th October a reserve corps of French ambulances was sent up to help the English section, and allow them a rest they sorely needed. Now and then a car had got stuck in the muddy holes; but neither a car nor a man had been hit.

There followed a period of a few weeks of local but sharp attacks by the Germans. The convoy was kept busy, though its activity was hampered by the continuous bad weather. In the mud of that desolate country the roads leading to the advanced posts became impassable. Horse-carts had to be used to bring the wounded to the farthest points which the cars could reach; and even the horses would sometimes slip and fall into pits of mud from which they could not be extricated. By 17th November the whole convoy returned to its base, sending out cars to be posted as near to the front line as was practicable. But the Germans were now making formidable attempts to retake the positions lost in the great battle. These were unsuccessful; but the fierce fighting caused many casualties. The conditions of transport for the wounded, owing to the rain and the mud, were miserable; it was so far for them to be carried, or carted, to the roads which were still practicable for the ambulances. The problem was tackled, and it was found that by making a long detour it was possible to get the ambulances up on the hills near the firing-line and to establish two new posts there. This was done, and the posts were kept in full activity, with narrow escapes from shelling by the enemy.

This ends the story of the Anglo-American Convoy, as originally constituted in October 1914. For in December a reorganisation of the foreign *Sections Sanitaires* serving the French armies was carried out.

The American members of the convoy left, to form a new, purely American section. The British members remained, and were now to be known as *Section Sanitaire Anglaise* 17.

On Christmas Day the unit was reinforced by the advent of a new convoy. This consisted of twenty ambulances, four lorries, a kitchen and a touring car. It had been presented to the British Red Cross by the Derbyshire and Nottinghamshire Coalowners' Association. This convoy now became Section 16.

The new section relieved the old convoy at once till January, when it was withdrawn to reserve.

A lull followed.

On 13th February the two sections were moved to another district. On the 18th they received orders to received orders to stand by, ready to start for an unknown destination at half an hour's notice.

Rumours were running along the front. There was in all ranks an air of tension and excitement; the sure feeling of a great blow coming from the other side, but uncertainty where it would strike, and what particular line was threatened. German aircraft began to cross the front, and dropped their bombs behind it. They were seeking to destroy the railways.

The omens were pointing to Verdun.

Well did the English sections acquit themselves in the unparalleled struggle which was now about to begin on the hills beyond that famous fortress. But Sections 16 and 17 were not the only English sections to play their part, and share in the incomparable defence. And before telling the story of what happened at Verdun, we must go back to 1914 and see what other units had been formed, and what work they had been doing.

The activity of the Friends' Ambulance Unit has by no means been confined to convoy work with the French armies. Hospitals at Dunkirk, Ypres, and other places; ambulance trains; hospital ships; recreation huts at Dunkirk; a preventive campaign against typhoid among the civilians of Flanders; relief and sanitary work in the destitute Flemish villages; these are some of the various enterprises which have occupied its overflowing energies. But here it is with the convoy service for the French wounded that we are concerned. The unit devoted itself to this work at a very early stage, and it occupies some two hundred of its six hundred members in France.

The unit is an unpaid voluntary unit of the Red Cross. It was formed at the outbreak of the war by members of the Society of Friends, is supported by Friends, and consists chiefly of Friends and others closely associated with them.

Everyone knows that the Quakers as a religious body have always held that war is wrong, and the use of force contrary to Christian principles. But the monstrous explosion that rent Europe in August 1914 was instantly seen to be no ordinary war. Old problems presented themselves in new aspects. Searching each his heart, and acting each on the command of conscience, the members of the Society came to no unanimous conclusion on the question asked with so much pain and perplexity, whether it was right to participate in this terrible struggle for the things most dear to free men, and, if so, in what form or in what degree. Our story is concerned with that large body of Friends who were determined to serve their fellow-men in the struggle, though resolved also not to be combatants.

On 7th September 1914, a camp was opened at Jordans, in Buckinghamshire, associated with so much of the early history of the Society; and here a group of eager young men began a varied and thorough course of training as a preparation for the ambulance work with the armies to which they looked forward.

But it was one thing to determine to serve at the front, it was another to secure the work desired. The Society of Friends has, naturally, no sort of relation with military officialdom, and its band of voluntary workers had, apart from their training in camp, no experience; they had neither connections nor influence to help them. But the will found a way. The pioneers of the unit chose for their motto, 'Search for the work that no one is doing; take it, and regularise it later, if you can.' In the first months of the war there was indeed plenty of such need and opportunity.

It was the sight of thousands of wounded soldiers arriving at the coast, having received little or no attention beyond a field-dressing eight to fourteen days before, and with pitifully small provision for their housing or transport, which decided the first emissaries of the unit, sent to France to prospect for work, that there was no need to seek further. Here was a gap which was not filled, and which their men could fill.

A hurried reference to the committee at home which was responsible for the unit brought the answer to go ahead.

In less than a week a little company of forty-three men and eight small ambulances were ready to start. They assembled at their rendezvous on the south coast on a day in late October. Some had come by rail, some by road. Many had had no time to take leave of their families. It was truly a going-out into the unknown; for the party did not know whether work would be given them, or where they would lodge on landing.

Early next morning, the unit started across the Channel; and almost immediately, without sound or warning, were plunged into the realities of war. Out of the mist, the shadowy shape of a great ship came into view. She was slowly sinking. It was the cruiser *Hermes*, which had just been torpedoed. All set to work to man the lowered boats, and for hours were busy saving the lives of the shipwrecked, hauling them from the water, pulling them up the steamer's side, or helping to restore animation. The steamer put back to land the survivors; and it was late in the evening before the unit reached Dunkirk.

It was the most critical time of the obstinate, massed, and furious attempts of the Germans to break through to the coast. The French wounded were coming back from the front in train after train. The congestion was extreme; and the railway sheds at Dunkirk were crowded with these poor sufferers, who lay there till their turn came to be taken farther back from the fighting-line. Meanwhile, there was no time to attend to them, or care for their wounds. Here at once, and on the spot, the Friends, at the end of their first day's journey, found the work they sought.

The sights, sounds, and stench in those dark sheds were their initiation, abrupt and horrible enough, into the world of waste and torment, death and mutilation, in which the Red Cross moves and has its being. But the members of the unit, fresh from home, and tired as they were, set to work with undaunted resolution, in spite of nausea and fatigue. Night and day they laboured, first continuously, then in shifts, while night and day fresh wounded arrived, to be heaped on the floor of the sheds in every phase of exhaustion, brokenness, delirium.

At last the pressure diminished. In a few weeks the regular *Service de Santé* had its disorganised machinery smoothly working again, and were able to take over the railway sheds from this unaccredited but so zealous and eager bands of workers which had suddenly appeared from nowhere. Much hospital work among the French remained, however, to be done, and of this the unit shouldered a considerable share.

This first experience taught the Friends that their cue was to be above all adaptable and elastic in their methods. Where a need called, and a gap appeared, there it was their place to be; and as soon as one urgent job was done, they must be ready to leave it for another.

The great desire of the unit was to obtain ambulance work at the front, and for this it was necessary to overcome prejudices against non-military volunteers. One of the unit, to whose vivid report these lines are much indebted, and who has since served the Red Cross with high distinction in Italy, wrote: 'At one time I counted that we were dealing with fifteen military authorities simultaneously; only five of whom could really help us, but any one of whom, if wrongly handled, could have blocked all our chances.'

Tact and perseverance carried the day. After a brief spell of work at Ypres, cut short for a time by the heavy shelling and temporary evacuation of the city, the Friends drove northwards along the front of the French armies, offering their services as they went.

At the village of Woesten, which was afterwards to become familiar as their parent station, they were warmly welcomed by a French evacuation hospital. Quarters were found for them in a school, where they speedily made themselves at home; and here the ambulance work of the unit with the French began in good earnest. The men were on their mettle, and worked devotedly, driving the cars under shell-fire, or by night and without lights, along the broken and pitted roads.

New stations were started, as requests for help came in: before long there were seven maintained at once. The most northerly was at Dickebusch. There were reinforcements from home. The unit doubled its numbers. The village of its first welcome, Woesten, became a distributing centre. The work expanded in every direction, as the men became more experienced; and during the great battles of Flanders in the closing weeks of 1914 the small fleet of ambulances covered more than 20,000 miles.

Towards the turn of the year the fighting gradually subsided, as the assaulting storms of the enemy attempts to break through to the coast were baffled and died down. The unit therefore withdrew its ambulance stations, one after another, and sought work more urgent.

The good work done had won the confidence of the French, and definite tasks were soon allotted by the authorities to the unit, which was now officially recognised. Another English Red Cross unit combined with it, and the large accession of good cars and drivers, now made over to the control of the Friends, greatly strengthened its resources.

In March 1915, cars from scattered groups were collected into definite convoys, and the *Sections Sanitaires Anglaises* Nos. 11, 12, 13, 14, and 15 were organised. No. 14 was staffed entirely by the FAU, and some of the other convoys were under officers belonging to it.

Some of these sections were kept in reserve at the base.

Most, however, were attached to various evacuation hospitals. The work done was cordially appreciated by the French, who wrote of the promptness, the regularity, and the unweariable never-faltering zeal of their 'excellents camarades.'

Towards the middle of April, Section 14, which had been kept in reserve at the base, received orders to report next day to the Algerian Division. This division held the northern part of the Ypres salient, with the Canadians next them on their right. Their line ran from the Yser Canal to a point just east of Langemarck. Duly reporting at Elverdinghe, the section found that it was to be responsible for the transport of the wounded of the entire division. After the impatience of inaction at the base, this great responsibility was inspiring. The accustomed routine of evacuation began. But in a very few days the men were to be put to a severer trial than any could have imagined.

It was the twenty-second of the month; a day of pleasant spring weather, with a hot sun and a light wind blowing steadily from the north-east. Evening was approaching, when, with hardly a moment's warning, fierce bursts of firing were heard, and the whole line was thrown into an unexplained confusion. The men of the convoy, working behind the lines, were met by a wild surge of Turcos and Zouaves staggering back from the trenches. They were ghastly to look at; they were coughing horribly; they could neither see nor speak. Numbers of them had dropped by the roadside and lay there overcome and insensible. And a strange, sickly, suffocating odour began to come down the wind, while the sky seemed to take on a greenish tint. It was the German posion-gas.

Astonishment at the apparition of the slowly advancing

greenish-yellow clouds, seen for the first time in the war on this pleasant April afternoon, had quickly been lost in the horror of the fiery fumes invading eyes and throat and tortured lungs. The Algerian troops had no defence against the agonising poison. It was as if some devil had been let loose among them.

The Second Battle of Ypres had begun.

The cars and men of Section 14 were wellnigh overwhelmed by the streaming mass of the victims of this new horror. Units were mixed up in an indescribable chaos. The resources of the convoy were all too insufficient for the moment. The men worked as they had never worked before, and for seventy-two hours most of them were to work without a break.

The French were being rapidly forced back all along the line from Steenstraate to Langemarck. On their left they had withdrawn behind the Yser Canal, and the enemy were pushing across it at more than one point. On their right, between the French and the Canadians, was a broad gap of four miles, through which the Germans were advancing. That the enemy never got right through was owing to the superb tenacity of the Canadians, who held on somehow, letting no troops win their way past them, till before the night was over the gap was, after a fashion, filled with reinforcements. Facing the gap was the chateau in which Section 14 had its headquarters; and on this night of terror and tumultuous confusion the battle rolled back almost on to the ambulances. Without a pause the cars drove to and fro, evacuating at utmost speed to the railhead and then returning, though each time the men knew that their posts might by now be in the hands of the enemy. Worse was to come. The gas attack was supported by a heavy artillery fire, and the railhead was driven farther from the front by the storm of shells; the horse-ambulance services, which had previously brought the wounded from the *Postes de Secours* to the motor ambulances, broke down under the strain; and at the request of the French this latter service was taken over by the English section. Little wonder that, in spite of continuous and exhausting effort, it was impossible to cope with the stream of asphyxiated and wounded. But during the next two days, though the battle went on with unabated fury, measures were taken to bring up new resources.

As we have seen, the other sections were working for evacuation hospitals and on similar service in the district. The actual disposition of these cars was entirely in the hands of the Friends' unit; and all of these that were available and could be spared were hurriedly summoned to help the Algerian Division. By the third day nearly forty cars were working, and enough drivers to form two shifts; so that each car could work continuously for twenty-four hours. An American section also sent some ambulances to help. By this time therefore the demands of the work could be met, exacting though they were. The long distance from the dressing stations to the railhead, and the constant shelling of the roads, added to the pressure and the risks.

From the French Command came messages of the warmest thanks and appreciation. '*Les voitures automobiles anglaises ont fait preuve d'un zèle, d'un courage et d'un dévouement, auquels on ne saurait assez rendre hommage.*'

No other single call of such overwhelming urgency as this of the Second Battle of Ypres was made on the unit for a long time. But its resources were taxed to the uttermost in other directions during this spring of 1915, as long as the fierce fighting continued. In no single instance was a call unfulfilled. Twice within a few days a complete hospital had to be removed. The organisation of the supply (for everything, including petrol, had to be brought from the base at Dunkirk) was at this time a difficult matter; but it never failed. At last the German assaults and the counterattacks of the Allies subsided, and Section 14 went to a well-earned rest.

During this lull in the fighting, a reorganisation was carried out. The British Red Cross withdrew a number of their cars and all their men; the remainder of the cars were placed in Sections 13, 14, 15, and the 'Section Parc'.

After work at various towns, Section 14 returned to the front on the extreme north of the line, at Nieuport, or what was Nieuport before it was shattered to bits – that little seaport long deserted by the sea, with the waste of high sand-dunes on its flanks, which before 1914 seemed of all places the most peaceful and world-forgotten.

Section 13 had all the work of Dunkirk Station, and the hospitals fed from it. SSA 15 was occupied with civilian work.

In the autumn, after a surprise inspection from the *Grand Quartier Général*, the unit was invited to come in under the revised scheme for reorganising the non-military convoys working at the front.

Under this scheme each section was to have twenty ambulances with attendant lorry, touring, kitchen and workshop cars and a motor cycle. Each section was to be attached to a division; it was to form an administrative unit in itself for the purpose of billeting, drawing rations, etc.; it was to have a French lieutenant attached to it, who would supervise and, with the unit's own *Chef de Section* or Commandant, be responsible for efficiency in working and for the exact execution of orders.

The generosity of the British Red Cross enabled the unit to accept this offer; and the sections were reformed on the prescribed model of the new scheme.

Soon after this, Section 13 was ordered to leave Dunkirk and to work for the French division holding the line between the Belgians and the British. To take its place at Dunkirk, what is called a '*Groupement,*' consisting of fifteen cars, was formed at the request of the French.

Our scene shifts from mud of Flanders and chalk downs of Champagne to the snowy heights and valleys of the Vosges.

About the middle of January 1915, there arrived at Bruyères – twenty miles or so behind the trenches – an English convoy, complete and perfectly equipped, sent out by the British Ambulance Committee. The committee, as we have seen, was brought into being by an Englishman, who felt that France, with her vast battle-line, must need more motor ambulances, and, having ascertained from official sources that the need was urgent, determined to procure her help from Britain. After negotiations with the military authorities in France, and with the *Union des Femmes de France* in London, a definite offer was made to form a British Committee: Monsieur Poincaré and Monsieur Cambon approved; the committee was formed and set to work in October. The French Ambassador and the British Ambassador in Paris became Vice-Presidents. Difficulties were encountered, as the ambulances were intended for work on the actual front, and the French authorities, conceiving perhaps that these civilian volunteers were elderly gentlemen of more leisure than activity, showed a wish to set them on evacuation work at the base. But objections were overcome, and before the end of the year two complete convoys, modelled on the pattern of the French Army *Sections Sanitaires*, were ready.

The first convoy, accompanied by the second, disembarked at Le Havre at the beginning of January 1915. The men were full of enthusiasm for their adventure, though none of them knew as yet anything about the work they were eager to be at, or the conditions they were to work under. Cordially received everywhere by the French, they arrived at Troyes, where, to their dismay, they found that the service allotted them was, after all, to be scattered about on a mild routine of evacuations. But a visit from the Chief of the Motor Staff at the *Grand Quartier Général* removed certain misunderstandings; and in a day or two the first convoy was on its way to the southern end of the Vosges. It counted itself fortunate in falling among a group of staff officers attached to the Motor Service who were as sympathetic and understanding as it was possible to be.

The second convoy was sent to Commercy, on the St-Mihiel salient.

The two convoys were to be known as *Sections Sanitaires Anglaises* No. 1 and No. 2.

Attention, in England at any rate, has been so much focused on other parts of the line in the West that the doings of the French in the Vosges have not been much described and are not perhaps too clearly remembered. It will be recalled, however, that at the outset of the war the French Command decided on an offensive campaign in Lorraine and Alsace. In the first three weeks of August there were some brilliant successes, and then came a marked check. The danger to the armies on the French left, driven back at Charleroi, prevented any following-up of the success on the right: and Mulhouse, which had twice welcomed the advancing French in its streets with extravagant rejoicings, was a second time evacuated. None the less, the gains achieved were important; they were kept; and a substantial strip of German territory was occupied.

The frontier for a good distance from Mont Donon, which is nearly opposite Strassburg, follows the crest of the Vosges southward as far as the Ballon d'Alsace at the southern end of the range, where the hills drop into the plain in front of Belfort. In January 1915, when the first English convoy arrived in the Vosges, two of the northern passes over the mountains were in German hands; but from the Col du Bonhomme southward not only were the passes held by the French, but their line was some distance beyond, and well inside the German frontier. They had advanced from the Schlucht Pass to the heights above Münster. They had descended the Thur valley from the Col de Bussang, and taken the town of Thann. They had established an advance post on the Hartmannsweilerkopf, a craggy mountain spur standing in the angle of the junction of the two rivers, the Thur and the Ill. During this month of January heavy fighting was still going on – the French still pressing down the valley of the Thur towards Cernay, and also farther south towards Altkirch and Mulhouse – when a tremendous snowstorm, lasting ten days or more, stopped progress on either side.

On its arrival, the first convoy was tried for several days on evacuation work in column, over rough ground, and up and down very difficult passes. The weather was wild, and the snow deep. During a strong but abortive attack on the Hartmannsweilerkopf, the horse-transport had proved very inadequate: it was twenty-five miles from the front to the railhead; and only one complete journey a day could be made. The cars could, however, do four or five, with far less suffering to the wounded. One half of the section was sent to the head-waters of the Moselle, under the Ballon d'Alsace, where it spent a strenuous three months, while the other half was kept equally busy behind the lines near the Schlucht Pass, where the Germans at one time nearly broke through. In this short period the men of the convoy had gained invaluable experience, and, though they had had no training in England, soon acquired the cohesion of military discipline. They had no accidents on the road, and never figured in the Orders of the Day for petty delinquencies.

The snow began to melt in March. The Germans were concentrating in the Sundgau, the plain in front of the Gap of Belfort, and the French apprehended an attempt to push through the Gap. The section was therefore reunited and sent to Belfort. But the threatened attack did not come off; and after a tedious time in the garrison town, the section was happy to renew its active service. It took part in two or three attacks at La Fontenelle north of St-Dié. Though the English public has heard so little of the Vosges fighting, these were big engagements. The work of the section was severe, and though the summer had come the rains continued, and the mud in the lower ground was as difficult for the heavy cars as the ice and snow on the hills in winter. Early in July the battle at La Fontenelle subsided, and the section retired to its original base to refit.

The French were so well satisfied with the first two convoys that they asked if more could be supplied. A third convoy was inspected before starting at Buckingham Palace by H.M. the King, on the 6th February, and shortly afterwards arrived in the Vosges, where it became Section 3. A fourth convoy reached France in June, and proceeded to the same part of the front.

During 1915 various changes were made in the organisation of the *Sections Sanitaires*. At first the number of cars in a convoy was to be twenty-five; then it was raised to thirty; then again reduced to twenty. When this last change was decided on, the British Ambulance Committee were able to create a fifth convoy from the surplus of the others; this became Section 5, and has always been, like Section 4, in the Vosges.

Early in September a new Army Order provided that each section should be attached to a division. Sections 4 and 5, though attached to divisions, have not been transferred from the part of the front which they serve, and therefore have worked with many divisions in turn. Sections 1 and 2, on the other hand, and Section 3, for part of the time, have been attached to particular divisions whose movements and fortunes they have followed. This has been the case with most of the English sections.

It was no light task that was required of the ambulance drivers on the mountain roads. The Vosges descend abruptly to the plain on the eastern side, though on the French or western side the slope is much easier. The general aspect of the range resembles the mountains of the Black Forest, which rise opposite to it, some thirty to forty miles away. Midway across the intervening plain, the Rhine flows northward from Basle, seen as a remotely shining band of silver from the heights on either side. The mountains are mostly covered thick with pines and divided by deep glens. Winter begins early and lingers late, and heavy snows are apt to block the roads and choke the upper valleys with their drifts. In thick snow on a dark night, when the zigzag roads up on the heights are slippery with ice, and lights have been switched off because the road is under fire, the limits of difficult driving are surely attained.

Spring had passed into summer, and the fighting in the hills and on the plain went on with little intermission. In June the village of Metzeral was taken from the Germans, and our ambulances were kept working at high pressure during the action. For the following month the French planned a big attack. As we have seen, one of their lines of advance had been from the Schlucht Pass down the valley of the Fecht, and they had gained the heights above Münster. But on the north of the river there was a mountain-spur, the last of the hills overlooking the plain of Alsace toward Colmar and the Rhine, which it was important, if possible, to win. This is the mountain called the Linge-Kopf, a massive, rocky promontory crested with pine-woods, which before the autumn were to be razed by ceaseless shell-fire to a stubble of charred stumps.

The attack began in late July. The nature of the ground made the operations singularly difficult. For six weeks the battle continued, furious stroke and counter-stroke answering each other, and at last died away in September, with little result but sanguinary losses on both sides.

The sections were attached to divisions of the famous Chasseurs Alpins. Nearly all the French regiments now wear the ' horizon-blue ' uniform, but the Chasseurs Alpins still retain the dark-blue uniform and Scotch bonnet, from which they have taken their name of *Diables Bleus*. The soldiers come from the mountain districts of France, and are hillmen born and bred; rather short of stature, on the average, but squarely-built, tough and active. Their fighting qualities are famed. The English convoys were proud to be associated with this splendid corps, and the men of the ambulances were on terms of cordial good fellow-ship with the soldiers.

Sections 1, 3, and 4 were all called on to serve in this attack. Section 3 brought the wounded down a steep zig-zag road, the corners of which were under direct fire from the Germans, from a large underground *Poste de Secours* high up on a mountain-side. For eighteen days and nights consecutively the men worked, without taking off their clothes. The whole convoy was on the road all the time.

The roads, worn and broken up by the incessant traffic of cars and motor lorries and mule transport, and bitten into by shells, became rough in the extreme. After heavy rain the mud was nearly knee-deep. Back-axles would break, or some other serious accident would constantly occur; and then the car would have to be towed home. Two spare cars had to be kept at the base, ready to start at a moment's notice. Scarcely a night passed without a summons coming to tow a car which had broken down.

Section I was working a little farther off, to the north. And their drivers had perhaps even greater difficulties to encounter; they had to work over crests of the Vosges by a road which previously was reckoned incrossable, and was extensively shelled. After the worst eighteen days the convoy was reduced from about forty cars to seven.

Section 4 had twenty-eight cars continually working high up on the mountains from a collection of huts in the forest to a little lake. The roads at that time were no better than mule-tracks, which the cars had often the greatest ado to climb.

The Germans were continually trying to block the moun-tain road by which supplies came up, and by which Section 3 carried down the wounded, by bursting huge shells upon it. Once they succeeded in blocking it for a short time, the seventeen-inch shells smashing up the rocks and tumbling them in a heap across the road. But even this did not interfere with our ambulance men's labours. Cars were sent round which brought the wounded down from above as far as the barrier. Other cars came up to the nearer side of it; and the wounded were quickly carried round and transferred from one car to the other. At one of the corners on the zigzag bends, directly under the fire of the German snipers, one man of Section 3 was killed and several more were wounded. To prevent repair, the Germans constantly burst shrapnel over the road. But in spite of everything the wounded were all brought down safely. And when one remembers how they were formerly carried, in springless carts, taking thirty hours to do what a motor ambulance accomplished in two or less, it is easy to imagine the incalculable value of an efficient service of automobiles. The protracted anguish of the long ride, with the constant result of septic poisoning, ended frequently in the loss of lives which are now saved by speed.

At the time of the block on the road, timely service was rendered by the motor-cycle side-cars which have been introduced on the Vosges front by the British Ambulance Committee. A track was somehow cleared for the side-cars, which were the first vehicles to go through the gap, and which brought the wounded to the waiting ambulances.

The first of the side-cars was delivered to the section in May 1915, and there are now twenty-three of them working over practically the whole of the Vosges front. The motor ambulances were a vast improvement on the former methods of transporting the wounded; but the ambulances could not go beyond the roads (such as they were), and serious cases were carried from the lines to the cars on stretchers by four men. The journey would be sometimes two or three miles, requiring eight stretcher-bearers. This method meant prolonged suffering to the wounded man; and the side-cars not only saved suffering, but released soldiers. At one post they enabled twenty-two out of thirty stretcher-bearers to be freed for other service. The machines have heavy tyres, with very low gears, and are able to go easily over the steepest and roughest of roads. The Alpine Posts or field hospitals on the Vosges front are now all served by side-cars. Garages have been made for them in specially constructed dug-outs. The cars go out to the first-aid posts, and bring the wounded into the field hospitals, where the ambulances collect them. Perhaps they have saved more lives even than the motor ambulances. The work of the drivers is hard and dangerous, day and night; all lights are forbidden, and to drive across a shell-hole, frequent in the rough lanes, means a disaster. The side-car section has served in the attacks on the Reihackerkopf, the Tête des Faux, the Violu, and other engagements; four of its members have received the *Croix de Guerre*; and some four thousand wounded have been carried.

In the autumn of 1915 Section 1, after a period of rest-ing and refitting, moved to a quiet sector in the northern Vosges. The Mayor of Bruyères presented them on their departure with an address of regretful farewell. The rela-tions of the English convoys with the French, civilians and soldiers alike, were, and continue to be, of the friendliest. The fact that this part of the front is remote has made the presence of the English uniforms all the more valuable as a symbol of the common cause of the Allies. And the men of the sections have always considered it as not the least of their functions to cultivate this friendliness. Sections 4 and 5 have been continuously in the Vosges from their first coming out; at least one sector has never been served, since that time, by any but British ambulances, and the men have become familiar figures of the countryside.

To turn aside for a moment from scenes of pain and bloodshed, let us take a glimpse at a Christmas festival in the Vosges at the end of 1915. In this case it was Section 4, to the Commandant of which occurred the thought of giving a party to the children of the town where the section was quartered. He consulted the Mayor, and arranged to call up the groups of children from two to seven years of age. The General of the Division came to hear of the project, and let it be known that if he were invited he should attend the party. It appeared, however, that a children's party after the English fashion did not approve itself altogether to the children's teachers and parents: they preferred a concert. So a concert was determined on, and a distribution of toys was to take place half-way through. The Town Hall was placed at the Commandant's disposal: but it was not an exhilarating interior: and someone suggested the theatre of the Casino, which had been closed since the war began. The theatre was applied for: it proved to be a chaos. Rain and snow were coming in through the windows, which had been smashed for months; the orchestra and the boxes were filled with straw, where soldiers had been sleeping, the seats broken and piled up on one another; on the stage, the prostrate scenery lay in a dingy heap. But what could not be done when the General was coming?

A word to the major of the garrison, and soldiers were soon putting the theatre ship-shape: in a few days it was ready for any festivity. The General invited his staff in his 'Orders of the Day.' There was no lack of musical gift forthcoming: professionals with a Paris fame were serving in the ranks and delighted to perform. On the first Sunday after Christmas, then, the theatre, swept, garnished, newly heated and newly lighted for the occasion, was besieged by eager crowds. A couple of hundred women and children were turned away in tears, for every corner was filled, and the whole house packed to suffocation. The auditorium was tumultuous with hundreds of children, vividly expectant. Eight volunteers of the section were on duty among the audience, putting chocolates into every open mouth at an interval in the concert. A little girl recited some lines of thanks to the Commandant, who led her on to the stage and made a speech in French. Then one of the Englishmen made his apparition through the prompter's hole as Father Christmas, and he too addressed the children in French; toys and cakes were distributed to the small guests as they filed past. And the General, among his staff, looked from the balcony, paternally applauding.

Such improvised festivities – for this is only an example – have helped perhaps to dissolve the legend of English people as *tristes*, unsocial egoists; they have left a pleasant remembrance that will last for years to come. The men of our sections interest themselves also in the life of the soldiers in the trenches. They play matches with them at football, and they help to form the little libraries from which books may be got to solace the dreary blankness of days in dug-outs. Friendships have been made that will not be forgotten on either side.

These happy relations are a solace for the routine of work which is often monotonous and rarely without hardship.

Sections 4 and 5 have moved about to various parts of the Vosges, sometimes in comfortable quarters, sometimes in draughty barns with straw for a bed, or in billets shared by cattle. The intense cold of the Vosges winter makes duty at out-stations on the heights a trying time; and the gigantic snowdrifts are often hard to get through. Motor-cyclists have on occasion been marooned for several days in the snow.

Section 5 was not formed till October 1915, after the attack on the Linge, and has not come in for any great engagement; but it has had plenty of severe and interesting work, and shared in many minor attacks. At one time it served the front between Dannemarie and the Swiss frontier, and evacuated to a distance of thirty-five kilometres from the lines; much of the work being done under fire and on dangerous roads. It has also worked high up on the snows of the Jura, in the bitterest winter weather, when the ambulances had to be pulled out of the snowdrifts by oxen. The front served by Section 5 is all, it is interesting to note, in the reconquered part of Alsace.

After the winter of 1915, Section 1 left the Vosges. We shall meet it again in other parts of the front. Meanwhile Section 2 arrived at St-Maurice, at the southern end of the Vosges, in December.

Section 2 had been busy on the St-Mihiel front since its first coming out in January 1915, doing the entire ambulance work for a whole Army Corps. In May it was reinforced by additional and more powerful cars, just in time for a German attack, during which all the cars were kept running for sixty hours on end. But after this a quieter time ensued, with occasional actions, and even these died down in the autumn. The summons to the Vosges, where an attack was preparing, was therefore hailed with joy. The convoy left Commercy on 1st December. The General commanding the Army Corps sent his band to play to them; he himself went round the cars, and shook hands, and thanked each of the men; and the convoy went off to the strains of the Marseillaise and the National Anthem.

Arrived at St-Maurice, the convoy found the winding road up the pass thronged with ammunition-carts, supply-transport, and all the preparations for a big action. The scene of the assault was to be the famous Hartmannsweilerkopf, the crags of which had already witnessed such desperate struggles. The attack began on 22nd December, and till the end of the year Section 2 was at work as difficult as it was dangerous, day and night. The roads were extremely steep, with sudden 'hairpin' bends; their surface was coated with ice and in places under incessant fire. With irregular food, and snatching what sleep they could under their cars, the men were a fairly exhausted band by New Year's Day. After this there was a less arduous spell, though intermittent fighting still went on. Then, on the 26th of February 1916 came an order to proceed with all haste possible to Bar-le-Duc. Though the section did not know it yet, they were bound for Verdun.

In the last month of 1914, a French volunteer Red Cross convoy, under the command of the Comte de K., was working at Amiens. This convoy contained two British members. One of them was a Scottish gentleman who had offered his car and his personal service to the French Government in November, and had himself taken his car out. He was afterwards, as we shall see, to take the leading part in organising a Scottish convoy.

Fighting was going on about La Boisselle; and the central *Poste de Secours* was in a village on the Somme. The wounded were brought to that point by stretcher-bearers, or wheeled on hand-carts, or carried in horse ambulances. Thence they were conveyed by the motor convoy to a town in the rear. But tourist cars had to be impressed to carry loads of wounded, even sometimes surgical cases after operation. The work of evacuation went on under pressure for three nights and two days continuously, in weather of driving sleet-showers and cold rain, till all the hospitals in the town were overflowing. There was a great scarcity of ambulances.

These experiences prompted the Scottish member of the unit, when his first leave came, to get more ambulances from Scotland. He had already taken charge of an ambulance sent from Glasgow, and now persuaded the Scottish branch of the British Red Cross to send out three more. Manned by volunteers, these were soon working hard, both at Amiens station, where the convoy was attached to the great evacuation hospital, and occasionally also at the front. It was the time of the brilliant offensive undertaken by the French between Arras and Lens, which captured Carency, Notre Dame de Lorette, and Neuville St-Vaast. But the extraordinary strength and elaboration of the German defences made the cost very heavy: and the work of the ambulances behind the front was correspondingly severe. Five more ambulances came out from Scotland in June 1915.

In this month the Comte de K. decided to form a new convoy for work in Flanders, leaving certain cars at Amiens. The Scottish volunteers, with their ambulances, accepted the invitation to join this new Anglo-French convoy, and arrived at Dunkirk on the 24th of the month. On the day before, the town had been heavily bombarded, and the men of the convoy had to clear their beds at the hotel of broken glass and fallen fragments. The general evacuation work of the district was assigned to them, with headquarters at Bourbourg. Trains arriving from the front were evacuated, and the wounded distributed among the hospitals in and about Bourbourg and Dunkirk.

In July all the British cars of the section, known as *Section Sanitaire Croix Rouge* 31, were removed to Bergues, now deserted of practically all its inhabitants. Here they were attached to a *Dépôt des Éclopés*, and collected the wounded from a wide area. In August, four of the cars were sent to the neighbourhood of Poperinghe, to work in conjunction with four of the French cars of the convoy. The ambulances were now getting considerably worn, though the mechanical skill of the drivers kept them going. On one day seven out of the eight cars broke down, but were all repaired by the morrow.

Towards the end of the year the pioneer of the group, whose original venture in taking his car out to France had led to the group being formed, returned to Glasgow to form a new complete convoy for the French front. His continued appeals for ambulances had borne fruit: the Scottish branch of the British Red Cross Society had given its support; a large number of cars was available.

The '*Convoi de l'Écosse*' was offered to the French Army by the Scottish branch of the British Red Cross, through the *Comité de Londres*, and was gladly accepted. The cars were all supplied by individuals or societies in Scotland. The drivers were volunteers, either over military age or exempted men. The ambulances arrived at Versailles on the

19th January 1916. There they were inspected, passed for service, and forthwith became Section 20 of the Sections Sanitaires Anglaises.

The eight cars of the Anglo-French group still continued to work in Flanders. Of the development of their work, as Section 20, we shall have more to say later on.

Meanwhile another complete section had been formed under the auspices of the *Comité de Londres*. This became Section 10.

Section 10 was formed in response to an appeal made to owners of cars to offer their cars and their services as drivers to France through the London (now the British) Committee of the French Red Cross. By degrees the unit was gathered together, and went over to France, where the members received a course of convoy training at the French Automobile base.

When ready, the section was sent to Picardy, and attached to a division. During the drenching rains of the early winter of 1915, it was occupied with the ordinary routine of divisional ambulance transport at the front. The bad state of the roads caused numberless motor troubles, but the work was carried on gallantly; the men were steadily growing more intimate with all its details and absorbing the spirit of their mission. They were soon to need all their resources.

At the beginning of 1916, Section 10 was moved farther down the line. It was stationed at Crépy-en-Valois, at Villers-Cotterets and in the Soissons district.

On 20th February the men of the section were quartered in a little farmhouse. Warning had reached them to be in readiness for a long journey eastwards; and they were now to start. Sections 16 and 17, of the British Red Cross, had received a similar warning, as we have told already, two days before, and started on this same 20th of the month. Rumours of impending attack by the enemy were in the air, and there was much speculation as to where he would strike. The general view was that it would be at Verdun. In those days, as the Commandant of Section 10 has recorded, Verdun was nothing more to them than the name of one of the great eastern fortresses like Belfort and Toul. Now it is a name spoken with a difference, and not lightly. It has become a legend and a symbol of France, of her bleeding heart and her victorious soul.

Eastwards the convoy made its way over the snow-covered country. It passed through Château-Thierry and Vitryle-François, and on through that devastated region, of which winter intensified the forlornness, to Bar-le-Duc. For two days it was billeted in out-of-the-way hamlets. At last came the order to report, the same night, at the headquarters of the 20th Army Corps. Surmise was now a certainty. The cars were headed for Verdun.

VERDUN

At midnight of the day on which it received orders to report at headquarters, Section 10 arrived at a certain barrack outside Verdun, which had been converted into a field ambulance. The battle had already begun, and the wounded were being brought in without ceasing. Long before dawn on the following morning the men of the section were up, and forthwith began work which went on without intermission till the 11th of March.

Who does not remember that sudden tension of feeling, that apprehension of a huge menace, which came on us all with the news of the first German blows on Verdun, and which so soon was to hold the breath of Europe and the world? To the wide public, this attack by the enemy, confidently launched in such force and mass, and so plainly meant to be irresistible, was overpowering in its unexpectedness. We had come to think of the Germans as definitely thrown on the defensive in the West; and now we were plunged back into a suspense that recalled something of what we had felt in the days before the Marne. And indeed, whatever might have resulted from the fall of Verdun, it still remains a marvel that the Germans did not succeed.

By the instructed, of course, this great enterprise of the enemy's was anticipated. Germany needed a victory; she expected a general offensive by the Allies in the summer, and she hoped, by luring them into premature attacks, to spoil it; if possible, she hoped to give France a mortal blow – at the least, to regain mobility. There were reasons, too, for choosing Verdun as the place at which to strike.

But into such questions we need not enter. Our business

is to try to see the battle as it appeared to our ambulance men, working behind the firing-lines.

The fact that France, who had given and suffered and done so much in stemming the onslaught of the invader while Britain was gathering together her forces, was now again summoned to meet so great an ordeal and again to pour forth the blood of her sons like water, made these Englishmen all the more determined to do their very utmost in her service.

Nothing yet had been seen or heard on any front comparable to the tempest of shells which was rained by the German artillery on the plateau beyond Verdun in those first days of the battle. Ridges, slopes, and hollows were battered with every kind of explosive, and the guns searched insistently for the roads, in order to destroy or dislocate the supply columns. Through this infernal hail the ambulances of Section 10 had to drive. Gas shells and lachrymatory shells were plentifully used, and sickening fumes were added to the nerve-racking roar of the explosions. By night the cars had to thread their way, always under fire, through the endless supply columns on the road. The sky pulsated redly with the glow from burning villages and from fires in Verdun itself. During the night of February the 24th snow began to fall; at dawn the frost was bitter, and the snow increased. The fighting continued furiously, and the pressure of the ambulance work never relaxed. It was not only at the posts that the cars had to collect the wounded. There were endless calls for them on the way, as the concentrated bursts of shelling struck among the moving troops on the roads and wooded slopes. The cars always brought down more than their full complement; they had sitting cases on the footboards, and even on the wings.

The men of Section 10 were working to *Postes de Secours* on the front, beyond Verdun; and they will not easily forget the crossing of the bridge over the moat into Fort Tavannes, nor what they saw in the woods upon the Fleury road. Fort Tavannes is on a spur just above the road leading from Verdun north-east to Étain. Next to Fort Tavannes northward is Fort de Vaux, and beyond that is Douaumont. It was on the 25th, the day the snow began, that the famous assault of Douaumont was made, and on that evening the German Kaiser, who had watched it from a hill within the enemy lines, telegraphed to Berlin his boastful message that the key of the last defences of Verdun had fallen into his hands. This, as we know, magnified the facts considerably, yet the moment was extremely critical.

During the four days of battle which opened on Monday, the 21st, four miles of ground had been lost. At the opening of the attack the French lines lay far beyond the ring of forts about Verdun; they were at a distance from the city of some eight miles in one direction and nine in another. Well inside the lines was that plateau of wooded ridges called the Heights of the Meuse, on which are the forts of Douaumont and Vaux and Tavannes. The plateau rises along the right bank of the Meuse, with Verdun sheltered behind it. On its farther side, facing Germany, it breaks abruptly down, with wooded ravines at intervals, to the clayey levels of the Woevre, green with marshes, gleaming with pools, and in winter deep in mud.

The French lines were out on the Woevre plain on 20th February, but by the 25th they had been withdrawn first to the skirts of the hills, and then still farther back on the plateau itself.

The first attack had been of irresistible momentum, as it was planned to be. A quite unheard-of number of heavy guns had been massed in the cover of the woods of the Woevre. Fresh troops were used for each successive assault, and each soldier (according to a German war correspondent) had been fortified to face the slaughter in advance by receiving a daily ration of three and a half pounds of meat. The mass of troops collected was enormous, and fourteen railway lines made it easy to bring up more.

The defence had none of these advantages. Besides the railway from St-Menehould to Verdun, which was exposed to easy bombardment, there was only a single narrow-gauge line, from Bar-le-Duc. The French positions had been prepared with consummate skill by General Sarrail in the autumn of 1914, but the trenches themselves and the communications had not been kept in fresh repair during the intervening period of quiet. The lines were held by Territorials, Chasseurs, and Colonial troops, in number only a third of the attacking forces, and during the first assaults they were reduced to odds of one to ten. They fought with superb tenacity, and the tactical skill of the command enabled them to exact an enormous price for every yard they yielded. But their own losses were severe enough, as the men of the ambulances working behind the lines had reason to know. Already the woods in the plateau were becoming splintered and shattered, and the roads broken up by shell-fire; but without ceasing the cars went to and fro with their loads of wounded. To Section 10 had fallen the high honour of being the first of the foreign ambulance sections to be sent to the front beyond Verdun. They had won the *Croix de Guerre* as a convoy, and now each car was entitled to have that cross painted on it. But on the lines behind the city there was equally vital service to be done. And we must return to Sections 16 and 17, which on 21st February had arrived at Baleycourt, a hamlet some three kilometres south-west of Verdun on the main road to Clermont-en-Argonne, and at once began to work from there to Clermont.

But already on the evening of the 21st, all traffic had to be diverted through a village to the south, so heavy was the shelling on the road and so many the holes broken into it. As for the railway to Clermont, it no longer existed. No lights could be carried on the cars, so the work of evacuation was doubly difficult. Next day two French sections were sent up to help the English sections. The hospital at Baleycourt was soon filled. The cars then transported the wounded on to field hospitals at Les Islettes, and other places in the Argonne. Occasionally they had to run into Verdun, which was already blazing in many places and was hit by frequent shells.

The congestion of traffic in the road was now extreme. The railway to Clermont and St-Menehould being now rendered useless, all transport came by road. This situation had been foreseen. Plans in full detail had been prepared a year before for supplying and doing all transport service for a large army on the right bank of the Meuse, independently of the railway, by road and motor lorry; and, as we know, this marvellously organised system, working day and night continuously, was the saving of Verdun. But with this press of traffic it may be imagined that the ambulance men found the work of evacuation as slow as it was difficult. Yet as the German attacks continued, day after day, with their tremendous violence, the stream of wounded increased. No sitting cases could be taken on the cars. All who were not on stretchers had to go on foot as far as Baleycourt, where they waited for motor lorries returning empty from Verdun. On each side of the muddy road, thronged with its unending chain of thundering motor traffic, the full *camions* going up to the city, and the empty ones coming down, these wounded trudged, helping each other along; and mixed with them were limping fugitives, old men, women and children, carrying what they could of their possessions, and too exhausted to turn and see the distant flames that from one point or another of the wintry landscape marked their burning homes. On this forlorn procession of wounded and homeless the heavy snow began to fall. Two days before, a whole suburb of Verdun had taken fire and was blazing. Movement on the road continued to be pitifully slow. The Commanders of the two English sections arranged with the Baleycourt hospital to have some large tents rigged up by the roadside. Here they supplied as many as possible of the wounded with steaming coffee, while they waited for a conveyance to take them on.

On the afternoon of the 28th February, the Germans began to shell the railway and road that ran by the hospital. By midnight the hospital had been entirely evacuated by the English ambulances, helped by the French, and the patients had all been carried to Vadelaincourt, another village farther off. And now welcome assistance arrived. Section 2 (of the B.A.C.) arrived – summoned from the Vosges – and joined in the heavy work on hand. Vadelaincourt was in a state of chaos. The hospital of sixteen hundred beds was full to the doors; and the wounded, famished and freezing, crowded everywhere. The roads were so blocked that it took sometimes two hours to go a single kilometre. Meanwhile an urgent telephone call from Verdun asked the English sections to clear eight hundred wounded from some barracks beyond the city which were being heavily shelled. Section 16 was sent up; but late on the 1st March the men, who had been working day and night continuously for several days, were so exhausted that the section was given a short rest; such men as could be spared from Sections 2 and 17 went up to relieve it and carry on the work. Yet Section 16, after a few hours' rest, resumed it next morning, and completed it by evening.

Meanwhile Section 10 was working its hardest along the road beyond Verdun and up to the advance posts, which one by one were being withdrawn nearer to the city.

The character of the battle had now changed. On 25th February the Brandenburgers took the fort of Douaumont, or rather its ruins, but the Germans could not establish themselves on the plateau, and they were driven back to the edge of it on the 26th by a brilliant counter-attack. General Pétain had arrived on the day before. Violent and massed attacks continued for a few days longer: but when the month ended it was plain that the original German plan of driving in the Verdun bulge by frontal attack had failed. A new plan was put into operation. This was to strike at either side of the bulge: and with March began the battles fought on the right flank for the Fort de Vaux, and on the left for the hills on the other side of the Meuse, the Côte de l'Oie and the Mort Homme. Local attacks of great intensity were made at intervals and at widely separated points. The work of the English sections varied therefore between spells of comparatively light service and spells of exhausting effort.

On 11th March Section 10 was relieved and went to

rest. The cars of the section were badly worn and strained. They had done good service, but the tourist-chassis of the cars was not really suitable for the rough conditions of the front. This was reported to the *Comité Britannique*, and new cars with truck-chassis were obtained through the generosity of the British Farmers' Association. The section was to return to Verdun before the summer was over, after a spell in the Forest of the Argonne. Meanwhile Section 16 was relieved on 30th March, and went to the base for a general overhauling of the cars; while Section 18, which had arrived in the course of the month, took its place in the barracks just outside Verdun.

  Section 17 continued to transport wounded from the Tent Hospital *de triage* at Queue de Malat to Vadelaincourt, Bar-le-Duc, and other places. The lightly wounded who had come down on foot went on to Bar-le-Duc in the empty lorries; but for men in a state of exhaustion, as they often were when they came down from the trenches, to travel some thirty miles in the lorries over rough roads without any food, was to run the risk of utter collapse. Section 17 therefore started a soup-kitchen, which from 6th March to 3rd April (when it was no longer required) was kept going night and day. Seventeen thousand bowls of soup were given out, and the timely refreshment made a great difference to the wounded and worn-out soldiers – in some cases perhaps the difference between life and death. The Minister of the *Service de Santé* visited the camp during March, and personally thanked the Section Commander for this service as well as for all the work the convoy had accomplished. The cars, which had all been through the Champagne battle of the previous September, were now exceedingly worn; and on 2nd May Section 17 was withdrawn for lighter work, and then sent back to the base for repairs. New ambulances were sent out, provided by the Dennis Bayley Fund.

During April the city of Verdun was again heavily bombarded, and Section 18 did fine service in bringing out under fire the men who were wounded by the bursting shells. So fierce was the bombardment, and so widespread, that shells began to fall about the barracks where the convoy was quartered. The section retired to tents a few miles farther back; and two days afterwards the barracks were hit by big shells causing many deaths. The German lines on both sides of the Meuse had by now been pushed nearer, and Verdun and its communications southward were the more exposed to the fire of long-range guns. But neither the Mort Homme on the north-west, nor Fort de Vaux on the north-east, nor the Côte de Poivre between them on the north, had yielded either to furious local assaults or to the general assault along the whole front by which, in this month of April, the Germans hoped to make good at last the failure of their first surprise attempt of February.

By now among the shattered woods young leaves here and there were breaking forth, as if no senseless havoc had been rained among their stems and branches – as if no infernal fumes had crept about their roots, as if no tortured men had moaned and expired beneath them in the darkness, frozen as they lay.

The French soldiers, conscious that all the world was watching their struggle, felt that they had proved themselves the better men. With the coming of spring and kinder weather they were more than ever confident that the enemy should never get through.

But though the gigantic battle had now subsided into a

sullen cannonade, with spasmodic onsets on the German side, set off by rapid counter-thrusts by the French, and though the struggle seemed over and victory won, the Germans had not yet brought themselves to own defeat; the lull was not to last; and a new struggle, as vast and terrible as the first, began in May, to reach a climax of intensity in the last days of June.

Section 2 had been moved up from Vadelaincourt on 16th April to a station at Queue de Malat, and was kept exceedingly busy till the 20th of June, during the terrific fighting of these two months, evacuating the wounded from the whole sector which it served.

On the left bank of the Meuse, the Mort Homme, Hill 304, and the wood and village of Cumières were taken by the Germans after incredible slaughter, before May was over. But on this side, the French line, though pushed back, held firm, and the Germans had gained nothing essential. On the right bank the enemy advance was more menacing. Douaumont had been taken by the French in a strong counter-attack on 22nd May; but the Germans recaptured it three days later. Then, thrusting with all their force and with massed battalions through the woods on the plateau, they isolated Fort de Vaux. Heroically defended for five days, the fort fell on 6th June.

More efforts were made, with a prodigious expenditure of shells and myriads of men. Thiaumont Fort, south of Douaumont, fell next; the village of Fleury, in front of Fort Souville, the last great outwork of Verdun, was taken, re-taken, taken again. But on the first day of July the French went forward and regained Thiaumont. It was on that same morning that the French and the English leapt from their trenches on the Somme and began their great attack. The thunder of the guns on the Somme soon had its reverberating effect on Verdun. Yet heavy fighting still continued; and Section 18 was so hard pressed with the work it had to do on the Verdun road, that Section 17, which had been repairing and refitting in a quiet quarter, was called up towards the end of June to assist it. Section 16 was also helping. The rain at this time was almost continuous, and the roads were slippery with mud.

In July, Section 16 relieved Section 17. On the fifth of this month Section I of the B.A.C. arrived from Lunéville. Its cars were lined up in the main street of Dugny; and in the cars the men ate and slept for three weeks. They were serving a *Poste de Secours* (taking turns with a French section) near Fort Souville, which had been the scene of such murderous fighting in June, and about which the battle still swayed, since the Germans made repeated and nearly successful attempts to take it. The road was encumbered at one place with a heap of dead horses; at another, batteries of 75's fired over the cars; it was often heavily shelled by the Germans, and the noise was deafening. Section 2, which had been for three weeks in the Argonne, returned on the 8th. Their division was on Hill 304; the *Poste de Secours* was at the foot of the hill, and the road to it, for some distance under the enemy's direct observation, was strewn with wreckage of carts, dead mules and horses, and with rolls of wire which got into the wheels and round the axles. Most of the cars were hit.

But the tide had turned; from now onward it was the French who, bit by bit, advanced, and the Germans who retired. The months between June and October were a time of obstinate struggle. And in August, Section 10, which had also been for a time in the Argonne, returned to

Verdun. Its division was the one which achieved the final recapture of Thiaumont Farm. Every night it had twelve cars at Verdun running up to the advanced posts until daybreak, when began the work of clearing from Verdun – still heavily shelled – to the different hospitals behind. The mist over the river between one and two in the morning was a great trial to the drivers. The section was cited in Divisional Orders.

On the 10th of this month, Section 2 moved to the right bank of the Meuse and evacuated from Fort Souville, and another *Poste* just below the summit of the hills, where shells shrieked continuously overhead.

During September Section 16 was moved down the Meuse, beyond Verdun, and took up the duty of transporting the wounded from Bras and Mont Grignon. Bras is a ruined village, which lay close to the German lines, exposed to machine-gun fire. Not a light could be shown, not a sound must be made, in moving the wounded from the *Poste de Secours*. Stretcher-bearers took the wounded on hand-carts down to the bank of the Meuse Canal at Bras; then they were put on barges and towed to Mont Grignon. The ambulances were stationed in that suburb of Verdun, and drove them thence to hospital. Section 17 continued at its post at Esnes, under Hill 304, and its duty was one of constant danger. The stretch of road from one ruined village to another was much exposed to shell-fire, and during the midnight hours, when the supply and ammunition carts were moving up, the enemy guns were always particularly punctual and attentive. The road itself was not only pitted with holes, but encumbered with wreckage of wagons,

Among the broken wheels lay dead and putrefying horses. It was difficult enough to steer the cars among these obstacles; but at night the confusion was thrice confounded. Endless transport columns moved up and down continuously, and among them pack-trains of donkeys, used to carry material of all sorts right up to the front lines, strayed across the road, in their wayward fashion; and all the while the shells were screaming and exploding in the darkness. The cars were often struck by flying fragments, but so skilfully were they driven that no serious accident befell them. After three months of trying service, Section 17 was withdrawn for a rest early in October. At the same time, Section 2 returned from a rest to Verdun, and took up the work of evacuating from Mont Grignon, in company with Section 16.

But in this month of October great preparations were toward. The French intended an advance in good earnest.

On the first of the month Section 18 returned to Dugny, behind Verdun, and evacuated the wounded from a *Poste de Secours* near Fort Souville. Both the post and the road to it from Verdun was under constant fire. One car standing outside the post was struck, and the front part completely destroyed.

On the 24th a powerful and swift attack was delivered; and with little serious loss, so well had the guns done their work, Douaumont was gloriously retaken.

During the days of this action, Section 16 and Section 2 shared the honour and the danger of serving their division side by side. It has been told already how the wounded were evacuated to Bras under close fire, and placed on barges on the canal below. This duty had only been carried out at night. But during the attack on Douaumont and the severe fighting which followed, it was necessary for Section 16 to carry it on by day as well. The weather was thick and rainy, the roads narrow and slippery, broken by shells and clogged by transport. But every car was kept on the road (no small tribute to the efficiency of the work-shop officer); and not only did the men perform their duties as drivers with unflinching courage and endurance, but some of them found time to re-dress great numbers of hastily bandaged wounds and to prepare and keep ready quantities of soup for the exhausted soldiers. Section 2 also did splendid service. Their work was particularly dangerous; nearly every car was hit, and one destroyed. Some of the drivers' lives were only saved by their steel helmets. The sections received the special thanks of the General.

With Douaumont recaptured, the French felt increasingly confident. A new stroke was prepared; and with a sudden onset, on 2nd November, Fort de Vaux was taken. The attack was so well planned that it was irresistible, and was carried through with but the slightest loss.

For a month and more there were desultory engagements; and then in December the heavy guns began their concentrated fire, and on the 14th the French advanced once more. This time the positions assailed were on the Côte de Poivre, which rises on the right bank of the Meuse, and at Vachereauville, a hamlet below it; immensely strong positions, held in great force by the Germans. It was wet and misty weather; but the French artillery was directed and controlled with consummate science, and almost before the enemy were aware that they were being attacked, the infantry were on them, and prisoners taken by thousands. Two days before the attack Section 1 arrived from Commercy, and Section 2 returned from another part of the line. Both served their divisions during the battle with unwearied devotion. There were many cases of trench feet among the Moroccans; for the weather was miserably cold and wet. Section 1 was split into two detachments, and had specially exhausting work in consequence. They won the *Croix de Guerre* for the convoy; and Section 2 (which had had four of its men wounded at Verdun) received eight *Croix de Guerre* for individual members, and one *Médaille Militaire.*

Section 17 also, which had been serving on the north-east of Verdun through the snow and sleet of November, moved, just before the attack, to Dugny, crowded at the time with the troops massing for action, and made shift to lodge in tents pitched in a sea of mud. The attack was so successful, and the German artillery reduced to such ineffectiveness, that the section's work was not so dangerous as had been expected, and few cars were hit. But the roads and all the countryside were now (as the Commandant of the British Red Cross Sections described in his report) in a lamentable condition. The bombardments of the German advance in the spring and early summer, and now the bombardment accompanying the French advance, had pounded old landmarks out of all recognition. Villages were now mere sites. Their former inhabitants would not have known their way upon familiar paths. The green forests that had crowned the ridges and filled the hollows of that wide, rolling plateau between the Meuse and the Woevre, would shed their leaves in autumn and renew them in spring no more. A few gashed stumps alone stood here and there on the flayed and pitted surface of the hills. It was absolute desolation. The bones of the horses of a gun-team lying beside the wreckage of a gun; skulls of German soldiers, fallen in battles of the spring, picked clean by the birds; boots, still casing flesh, sticking up from the earth that had buried a man;

all kinds of pitiable, mouldering wreckage made a region of pestilential ruin. In such charnel scenes were stationed the *Postes de Secours*, where the English ambulance drivers waited for their cars to fill with wounded, in dug-outs where the rats disputed possession with them, sometimes 'as large as puppies.'

Section 2 left the Verdun suburb where it was stationed during the last battle, towards the end of December 1916. Section 17 moved yet farther to the east of Verdun, and in the new year, after a brief rest, returned to the front near St-Mihiel. Section 1 also left Verdun in January 1917. Section 18 continued work in the near neighbourhood of Verdun for some months; Section 2 also returned there and served its division till the end of April 1917. On that date, Section 18 moved up beyond Verdun to a new *Poste de Secours* at the Côte de Froide Terre, one of the heights of Meuse. At this point the French had again advanced and taken the German positions. At short intervals Section 17 moved on to new posts on the Heights of the Meuse beyond Fort Tavannes, and at the end of May had extended their service to a yet more advanced post at the Vaux Pond, on a road which till then had been thought too dangerous to be used. Early in June the service was extended beyond Bras to a point not much over a thousand yards from the new German lines, and the wounded were carried straight back to Verdun and beyond on the ambulances, without being transferred to barges on the canal, as before.

After a month's rest the section came back to Verdun. Section 10 was also there. It was early in August. A new great attack by the French was preparing. And now the two Commanders of Section 17, English and French, being intimate with all the roads on the front allotted to their division, proposed to the General to take the ambulances up to two posts so far advanced that hitherto no cars had gone so far, and the wounded had always been carried down from them by stretcher-bearers. But manifestly if the cars could get there, the wounded would be brought down much quicker; and, though the roads were under more or less constant fire, permission was given.

On 20th August the attack was launched. The positions to be stormed were the Mort Homme and Hill 304 on the left bank of the Meuse – heights which had cost so many thousands of lives in the preceding summer – and the Talon, Hill 344, and Beaumont, on the right bank. These positions were all that were left of the German gains since their first overwhelming assault in February 1916. They had been made into fortresses of immense strength. With their masses of men and guns, they seemed impregnable. But after eight days of a terrible cannonade from massed artillery, the French infantry sprang forward. Nothing could withstand them. On the first day the Mort Homme fell; and one after another the impregnable positions were carried.

Section 10 again distinguished itself during this attack by its splendid work. On their right, Section 17 kept up its service for two days and nights continuously to the two advanced posts on the heights, though gas-shells with their suffocating fumes as well as shells of every kind were rained upon the roads. After the first day's advance, Section 17 pushed up to a new post in a quarry which the day before had been a German First Aid Post. The wounded were thus saved nearly three miles of stretcher-bearing, and in honour of the section's enterprise the quarry was named the Quarry of the English. After the attack the General sent an officer to thank the section for their services, and to say how the French rejoiced to have their English comrades serving with them.

During September, powerful counter-attacks were made by the Germans on the positions they had lost. Section I was now once more at Verdun and found the roads, up and down ravines and over ridges, worse than in any former experience and more heavily shelled. Beyond Fleury village, the very site of which was obliterated, even the stumps of the trees had been shorn from the crests of the hills. One man was struck by a shell, four others were gassed (seven more had been wounded already in an accident) and the cars suffered severely. It was the hardest and best work the convoy had ever done.

But all these attacks failed of their object. On the 26th August 1917, the French line was substantially restored to what it was in February 1916. The wheel had come full circle. The most tremendous and bloody battle in the history of nations had been fought: myriads of German lives had been given, myriads had suffered, and in vain. The arrogant and eagerly anticipated hopes of a people and a dynasty were buried in that vast grave of sacrificed nameless men; the green forests had been blasted from the hills; thousands of widows and orphans wept, and no one heard them. This was the end.

It was not four years since the Crown Prince, the hero appointed to victory at Verdun, had confided to Mr. Gerard's American friend that he meant to have war 'just for the fun of it.'

AND AFTER

So far we have confined our chronicle mainly to the doings of the sections when called on to serve during important battles and engagements. But if these are the times which test every faculty, and exact every ounce of endurance, the service of the members is equally indispensable in times when, as the bulletins tell us, there is 'nothing of interest to report.' On the quietest of fronts men are always being wounded; and there is continual evacuation work to be done to and from hospitals behind the lines.

Whether a section comes in for a frequency of exciting spells or not, depends on whether it is attached to a 'holding' or an 'attacking' division. Hence some of the English sections have had more, and some less, than their share of the action and danger which all are keen to face. But whatever they are called on to do, whether it be the monotony of routine work or the arduous nerve-strain of day-and-night exertion during a great battle, they work with a cheerful will. Just because they are volunteers, they will take risks that the regular convoys prefer to avoid.

The least interesting kind of work, useful and necessary as it is, is that of evacuating trains, field hospitals, or evacuation hospitals at the railhead. There are usually outlying hospitals to be served, and this work involves long runs.

At the front the normal routine is as follows: Regimental stretcher-bearers carry the wounded from the trenches, or the places where they have fallen, to the *Postes de Secours*. These are placed as close behind the firing-line as is practicable; it may be two or three hundred, or as much as two or three thousand yards. There the wounds are roughly dressed. The wounded are then sent on to a *Poste de Triage*, where they are sorted out, and, if necessary, have their hurts re-dressed. The lightly wounded are sent from the Triage to a Field Dressing Station, whence they can return to the front as soon as they are well enough: more severely wounded are sent to the nearest Casualty Clearing Station; the very badly hurt are sent to a Field Dressing Station till well enough to travel farther.

From the *Poste de Triage* backwards all the work is done by the *Section Sanitaire* of the division. And now the ambulances of the section almost always work the whole way back from the *Poste de Secours*. It has been told how at the time of the first gas attack in the Second Battle of Ypres, the service of horse ambulances which brought the wounded from the *Poste de Secours* broke down; and a section of the F.A.U. was among the first to replace the horse ambulances, and the '*brouettes*' or light hand-carts which were also used, with the far swifter automobiles. The roads are not always practicable for these; but the English sections have shown a fine spirit of enterprise in pushing up their motor service as near the firing-line as possible, as during the last of the Verdun battles; and in the difficult mountain-paths of the Vosges, by starting a section of motor cycles.

As the drivers of English sections rank as privates in the French Army, they receive the regular pay of five sous a day and army rations, which are supplemented out of mess funds. Cooking is done in the roomy and well-equipped *camion cuisine* or kitchen lorry. The workshop cars are fitted up with lathes and a variety of machines which enable them to tackle any kind of repair.

Billets are found in huts, tents, dilapidated cottages, or

ruined farms. Though many of the volunteers are men of middle age, there has been remarkably little illness among them. And in spite of a number of casualties, the good fortune of the sections has often seemed almost miraculous. More than once or twice a post or billet just vacated has been blown to pieces; and the story we have told is testimony to the storms of shell-fire through which they have worked for days and nights, and survived.

And now let us return to the beginning of the year 1916, just before the First Battle of Verdun, and see what was happening on other parts of the front, and what new developments had taken place among the English convoys.

In the Vosges, though little has been heard in the bulletins of the fighting, Sections 4 and 5 of the British Ambulance Committee continued their admirable and difficult work, on relations of ever firmer friendship with their French comrades.

During 1916, various sections were working on the front in the region of Lunéville, of St-Mihiel, in the Argonne, in Champagne, and on the Somme, as well as at Verdun.

In the extreme north, a number of British convoys were working for the French. At Nieuport, the ambulances of the Munro Corps, the story of whose aid to the *Fusiliers Marins* during the defence of Dixmude has been told already, continued their evacuation work. The number of cars was increased from six to nine, with a motor workshop and a small lorry. In June 1917, the British Army took over the sector, and the corps, after a few weeks' rest – the first it had had since September 1914 – joined the French forces stationed between the British and the Belgian armies. It took part in the actions of the late summer and autumn of 1917, when the French co-operated with the British in their great offensive in the north of Western Flanders. One of its cars was the only ambulance to cross the Yser Canal during this campaign, and to travel over a great part of the country so recently held by the enemy.

At the end of October, owing to the loss of old members and the difficulty of recruiting new ones, it was found necessary to disband the corps. It had had over three years of active service at the front. Several of the members had received the *Croix de Guerre*, and all those working in France on October 1917 were again mentioned in des-patches. When the corps left, the *Médecin-chef* of the army to which it was attached, wrote to express his regret, his gratitude, and his esteem.

To the Friends' Ambulance Unit, also, the Flanders plain had come to seem a second home.

At the end of 1915, it may be remembered, Section 13 left Dunkirk, and all the work connected with Dunkirk station, and the hospitals centring on it, devolved on a *groupement* of fifteen cars now formed to take its place.

Section 13 was stationed for more than half the year 1916 at Crombeke, a hamlet midway between Ypres and Furnes, while Section 14 had its headquarters at Coxyde, a village beyond Furnes, just on the border of that strange region of the Dunes – high hills and hollows of blowing sand – which divides the Flemish pastures from the sea. While it was here, two of its members were unfortunately killed. But at the end of August, Section 13 departed for the pleasant woods of Compiègne – a two-days' journey. And a few months later, Section 14 left their home on the coast for the first time, and travelled southwards, to shift from one uncomfortable billet to another in the region of the Somme, a world of rain and mud.

We shall hear of these sections again. Meanwhile all that was left of the F.A.U., in its old area, was the *groupement*. This continued its work at Dunkirk till September, when a new full section was created, for which it supplied the nucleus. The new section is known as Section 19. On its formation the *groupement* suffered a temporary shrinking, but after the quiet of the winter months regained its normal strength. Its work is carried out from four centres, the most important being an evacuation hospital (sometimes hit by shells or bombs), where sick and wounded arrive direct from the front, and where it has cars on duty night and day. It has been kept very busy, and has nearly rivalled the records both for distances run and patients carried, of a full convoy.

From September 1916, when it was formed, to midsummer 1917, Section 19 remained – with an interval at Dunkirk – working on the coast at Coxyde, where Section 14 had been before. It is the most northerly sector of the whole Western Front – a country where floods are apt to invade the floors of billets, and occasional sandstorms block the roads and bury the cars in drifts. Such incidents diversify the monotony of routine. Gas attacks, both by the French and by the Germans, with heavy shelling, were the chief events of this period. Towards the end of June this sector was taken over by the British. Section 19 went into *repos* with its division, but returned to the front in early August, 1917, during deluges of rain; and the successive great attacks by the British, in which the French co-operated, gave it plenty of work to do, though spells of quiet intervened. Early in October, its division took part in a forward thrust in front of the Forest of Houthoulst. The men were warned overnight to have their cars ready by

3am. As the cars were parked in a field, it took the greater part of the night to get them on the road ready for an immediate start. By seven in the morning the wounded were coming back to the post. The post would have been moved farther up after the advance, had the state of the ground made it possible; but nothing could have got the cars over the sloughs and swamps and flooded shell-pits. Numbers of young German prisoners were requisitioned to help carry the wounded over this chaos of mud and water, and, famished though they were, did the work well.

A little later the section returned to its old quarters and its old division on the coast. During its first year of existence it had been only absent from the front for fifteen weeks.

Besides the *groupement* of the Friends, there has been another *groupement* working in the Dunkirk region. This is the *Groupement Croix Rouge* of the *Comité Britannique*, the nucleus of which was the British element in the Anglo-French Convoy, of which an account has been given. The *groupement* was formed at the end of June 1916; it consisted of eight cars, afterwards increased to eleven, with eleven voluntary British drivers. Till December of 1916 it worked in the Boesinghe sector, between the Belgians and the British, and took the wounded from the trenches to a hospital at Rousbrugge, and from there to base hospitals behind. The men had a hard and dangerous time during a formidable gas attack by the Germans in August, but it performed its duties with fine spirit, was mentioned in despatches, and won the *Croix de Guerre* for several of its members. The sector was taken over by the British, and for a few months, after a rest, the *groupement* worked through bitter weather and frequent air-raids at Dunkirk. Then it went back to the sector in which Section 19 was working, and when that, too, was taken over by the British, returned to Rousbrugge. In August 1917 the old ambulances (gifts from generous donors in England and Scotland) were replaced by ten new G.M.C. cars, a lorry and a workshop car, presented to the *Comité Britannique* by the Scottish Coal-owners, the National Union of Scottish Mine-Workers, and the Scottish Branch of the British Red Cross. With these cars the *groupement* has done admirable service. It helped Section 19, among other occasions, during the attack we have just described.

This *Groupement Croix Rouge* stands in a sort of parental relation to the Scottish Convoy, Section 20 – also under the *Comité Britannique* – which we left at the time of its first arrival in France at the beginning of 1916. Its destination was Riquebourg, in the region of Compiègne; and within half an hour of its arrival it was working for its division. Accommodation was scarce; the room allotted for eighteen men did not allow of all lying on the floor, even on stretchers. Some space, however, was found in a cellar. The ground was deep in snow, and drivers had often a heavy task to dig their cars out of the snow and mud in the morning, for they were parked under the trees in the grounds of the château. On 21st February, the day of the first assault on Verdun, the section was moved to take over the service of another division. This was the division of General Marchand, who expressed his pleasure at having with him a British convoy. Here the front was lively, and the cars were out night and day, under frequent shell-fire. The section was complimented on its perfect regularity in answering calls and on arriving always at the posts in the minimum time allowed. Towards the end of June, the section was moved to Western Champagne, and instead of divisional duty on the front, undertook general Army Service. For this purpose it was divided up into small detachments, and did all kinds of evacuation work to and from a large number of widely scattered places. The cars were distributed over an area of something like a thousand square miles. Needless to say, the maintenance of the ambulances in good trim night and day, and the conveying of their supplies, etc., demanded careful planning and a great deal of sustained effort. After seven months of this service, more arduous than exciting, all the cars were gathered in under orders to leave. It was near the end of January 1917, and the severe weather was at its bitterest. Frost is no friend to motors; and with the thermometer some degrees below zero every night, it was impossible, with the most anxious precautions, to prevent radiators from springing leaks and engine-casings from cracking. Even warm water poured into protected radiators would freeze before circulation took effect. After a short rest the section took over the service of a division at the front, just at the centre of the scene of the first battle of Champagne in September 1915. A detachment was kept in continuous work at Suippes.

A second battle of Champagne was preparing, and troops were massing behind the lines.

It was still wintry when, in the first days of April, Sections 13 and 14 were moved to stations on the front between Rheims and Suippes. For two months Section 13 had been in the Argonne, and Section 14 at Châlons. A little earlier, Section 16 had been brought up from near St-Mihiel to the same front. Section 1 arrived from Verdun on the 13th of the month. Section 3 was posted near the Butte de Mesnil. Section 10 was posted near Section 20, but farther to the east.

On Monday, 16th April, a great offensive was launched between Soissons and Rheims. On the following morning the signal for attack was given on the east of Rheims, over a front of near ten miles, the front which the English sections were helping to serve.

For a full week the prelude of artillery had been thundering without intermission, and with a violence that seemed fantastic. The face of the landscape was pounded out of shape. Here, as in the battle of September 1915, was the same desolate country, with frequent patches of fir, the same powdery chalk soil, slimy after rain. And on the Tuesday, when the French infantry sprang from the trenches and went forward, the morning was raw and gloomy, with squalls of sleet which turned sometimes to rain, sometimes to snow. The German lines were in positions of great natural strength, on a range of hills, the Moronvillers Heights, which overlooked the ground below, so that every movement of the French could be plainly seen. The lines, too, were held in great force. Nevertheless, they were taken.

The highest national hopes had been built on this attack. Unfortunately, they were not destined to be fulfilled except in a very partial degree. But the first onrush was splendid. From Mt. Cornillet eastward a line of heights was carried. But on the left, where the enemy were entrenched in a great wood, strong resistance was met and the French advance was held up. The troops that had gone forward on the right had to be brought back to keep the line.

Of the English sections, perhaps Section 13 had the most dangerous duty to perform. The *Poste de Secours*, from which they had to bring down their wounded, was in a wood, on the left of the line, where the attack was least successful. The *Poste* itself was continuously bombarded; so was the whole stretch of road down which the cars had to run; so was the village to which they brought the wounded. The stranding of some 'tanks,' near the cross-roads where the cars waited, attracted the enemy guns' most earnest attentions. 'It was not unusual in passing up and down to find sentries, who had been passed an hour earlier, lying dead at their posts, and the road in places blocked, with dead convoy horses and some of their drivers.'

The night before the attack, one of Section 13's cars was hit three times in succession by shells, absolutely smashed and burnt: almost all the cars were struck by splinters; yet no one was killed, though two men were wounded, one severely. Section 3 had like experiences; five of its cars were hit, and the men suffered from the gas fumes.

Section 1 was at first called on to work wherever occasion demanded, as its division was split up and used as reinforcements. For a day or two the cars were lined up in the middle of the French batteries, and the men had exciting times. But on 25th April, Section 1 moved a little farther east (their old quarters being bombarded, and many killed, an hour or two after they left them), and till the middle of June they were working up to *Postes* in the fir-woods in front of the heights called the High Hill and the Hill Without a Name. They were fortunate in escaping without casualties, but won coveted distinctions from the General in command.

Section 16 served a *Poste de Secours* in a village, as well as another *Poste*, much farther advanced, in the woods. It fell to them to be frequently bombarded with gas-shells; but, though one of their men was badly gassed, the poisonous fumes did not prevent them from going cheerfully to and fro upon their duty. Section 14 and Section 20 worked side by side farther to the east on the line of attack. The General of the division to which Section 14 was attached, wrote later to congratulate it, and to thank the officers and men for their '*precieux concours*,' the regularity of their service, their coolness and devotion. 'The wounded French soldiers are grateful to their English comrades for having brought them such swift and efficient help.'

No less praise was given to Section 20. They too had the gas to fight, and were forced to abandon several of their cars in a cloud of gas during the night and bring them in in the morning. The long frost broke during these days of battle; much rain fell, and the roads were in a state of dissolution. Nevertheless all the wounded were brought back safely. The bombardment was at times terrific. The headquarters of the section was a ruined farm. A six-inch shell came through the roof of the shed in which their cars were stalled; and though it did not explode, it brought an iron joist tumbling down on the top of one of the cars, and then crashed through the engine of another car alongside. Had it burst, many of the men, who were working in the yard, would have been blown to bits. At the *Poste de Secours* the section was less fortunate. Here a wheel of a waiting car was struck off by a shell, and its driver was killed. He was a boy of seventeen who had volunteered for service in our own army, but had been drafted out when his age was discovered. Not to be baulked in his desire for action, he joined the Scottish Convoy. He had been with it only three weeks, yet had already earned the highest praises. But all the section did their duty with conspicuous bravery, and several of its members won the *Croix de Guerre*.

Section 10 was posted a little east of the battle front, but during the days of the attack they were called on many a time for special efforts.

About the middle of May the French went forward again, and captured the whole of the hills which were still in the hands of the enemy; and Section 2, which had come up from Verdun, served its division during the action, winning Army Corps 'citation' and *Croix de Guerre* for four of its men.

There is much more that might be told in detail about the doings of the various convoys. But enough has been described to enable the reader to picture the kind of experience which is theirs; the great battles and campaigns in which they have borne their part; the trials of mud, rain, and snow, besides the assiduous attentions of the enemy's artillery – bursting shells and choking gas – through which they must keep their cars going and in good trim; the cares of sensitive engines; yet with all this the satisfaction of doing good service for that splendid Army of France to which for the time they have the pride of belonging, of making firm friends with their French comrades, and of saving many a life by their promptitude, skill, and endurance.

But our tale is not yet complete; for we have not yet made mention of another convoy of the French Red Cross, which serves, not in France, but in the Balkans.

In October 1916, the *Comité Britannique* received a request for a motor ambulance convoy from the *Mission de Co-Ordination des Secours aux Armées d'Orient.* The Balkan Convoy was at once planned and soon brought into being. When complete, it consisted of fifteen ambulances, a staff touring car and workshop and repair car, manned by twenty-eight British voluntary drivers and mechanics. By the New Year, all was ready, some tons of stores included. During January the convoy was stationed in Surrey, learning perfection by practice, and at the end of the month was reviewed in Hyde Park by the French Ambassador.

On 3rd March 1917 the convoy arrived in Salonika Bay; and a few days after the whole unit was in camp outside the town. On the 12th the start was made for the front. On the second day Ostrova Lake was reached, and on the third Banitza. Here the convoy divided. Eight cars went to Fiorina, the rest to Slivica, close to Monastir. From Slivica, well up in the firing-line, the wounded were conveyed to Sakalevo, fifteen miles away; and from Fiorina to Exisson. For its good work and speedy transport of the wounded, the convoy has been warmly thanked by one of the chief medical officers of the Eastern Army. 'Your section,' he wrote, 'has been not only useful, it has been indispensable.'

Later in the year the convoy was reinforced by more cars, and by fresh drafts of voluntary drivers.

Among the drivers of the Balkan Convoy was a young Irishman, who had vainly tried to enter the British Army, but had been rejected for ill-health, and who died at Salonika. In his last letter he wrote:

> The risks, as days go by, seem of smaller and smaller account. I miss many, very many of the little luxuries of home, but I have enough and to spare. We are all so prone to put our own selves before the part – and it isn't a big one – we are playing in stemming the tide of human suffering that never seems to ebb...
>
> While in the main we are happy, we never cease to talk of home. Daily we conjure up what we shall do when that great day of peace shall dawn, the hours

we shall laze in the morning between sheets of snowy white, the meals we shall have... the visits to our old haunts. There is much to do in the meantime, work which will daily bring us near to suffering and self-sacrifice, and teach us perhaps some lessons in unselfishness and bring us nearer to finding our souls. On the whole there is renewed courage out here, and the hope of brighter

The letter ends abruptly, for the writer's hand was cold. In the words of this young ambulance driver one recognises the fine essence of the voluntary spirit, by which the work of the Red Cross is animated and inspired. Disguised it may be by the grumbling which is our cherished English prerogative, and rarely expressed in language, it is there; and with it goes the readiness to answer all calls, to refuse no service, whether in the bond or no, to acknowledge no defeat. 'What I like about you,' said a French officer to one of our convoy leaders, 'is that you will go *anywhere!*'

It remains to say something of the convoy work of English women. The First Aid Nursing Yeomanry Corps (sometimes familiarly known as 'Fanny' and more affectionately spoken of than the armed and intimidating 'Dora') was originally raised in 1909 and was trained on the lines of the RAMC training for stretcher-bearers and orderlies. All members of the corps are volunteers. Since the out-break of the war it has done a great amount of varied and valuable work for the Belgians and the British as well as for the French, some of it of a pioneer character. From October 1914 to October 1916 the corps maintained a hospital for Belgian wounded at Calais. Associated with this was a Belgian Convoy, with about twenty women drivers, which has on emergencies worked for the French wounded. These occasions were rare during the first two years, but have been more frequent since 1916. The convoy has also undertaken the work of collecting the wounded during the bombardments of Calais from the air and from the sea. During 1917, especially in the autumn, these were frequent and severe; and the promptness and intrepidity of the drivers have won warm praises and thanks from the Governor of Calais. In July of 1917 the Commandant of the Belgian Convoy made a formal offer of a FANY Convoy for the French Army. This was accepted, and in August she was asked to send a convoy of twenty drivers to Amiens. Drivers were collected, and the convoy set to work, under a French section, this same month. At Amiens there was no lack of work, including much night service. The cars were old and out of condition; but the French Commandant of the '*Région*,' seeing how the members of the FANY cared for their cars, provided new ones. The convoy was settling to its duties when in September it was ordered to move from Amiens, and was transferred to Villers-Cotteret, and thence to Château-Thierry. In November another convoy of ten drivers took up work at Épernay, where it is attached to the evacuation hospital. Yet another convoy is to work at Châlons.

An independent unit of women-drivers, known as the Hackett-Lowther Unit, was founded in August 1917. These Englishwomen draw soldiers' rations and form a military unit like the sections whose work we have been following; and, though they do not work on the actual front, they do valued service in transporting the wounded to and from evacuation hospitals and stations on the railways. They drive by night and by day, wherever they are sent.

Lastly, over and above the work of the convoys, it should be realised that there are some three hundred British cars serving various French hospitals, independently, dispersed all over France.

If now we resume for a moment that aerial vantage-point from which we began, we shall seem to see, scattered here and there along those hundreds of miles of the French front – from the wind-blown dunes of Flanders to the rocks and pines of the Vosges, in the defaced valley of the Somme, the forests of the Argonne, the chalk-downs of Champagne, the fire-scorched Heights of the Meuse – little companies of Englishmen with their grey Red Cross cars, driving the wounded to train and hospital, or going up to the posts where the guns are flashing and destroying. It is not they who will magnify their efforts; they have seen, they know, what the soldiers of France endure. But they have woven into that heroic stuff a bright thread of English comradeship. They know that they also serve.

THE HOSPITALS

HOSPITAL SUPPLY DEPOTS: AND THE FRENCH WAR EMERGENCY FUND

We propose to describe the hospitals in the order of their foundation. But before launching on the story of what has been done for the French soldier by our hospital workers in France, let us try to complete our survey of what has been done in Britain; for supply, as every one knows, is as important as the firing-line.

In writing of the activities of the *Comité Britannique* we noted that, besides sending out supplies on its own account, it forwards every day consignments of supplies of all kinds needed by the hospitals – the purely French as well as the Anglo-French – which have been made or collected in various parts of the country and are sent through the *Comité* to France. Where do these supplies come from?

All over these islands, very soon after the war began, voluntary workers banded themselves together to form Working Parties and Hospital Supply Depots and devoted all their time, or as much of it as they could spare, to making things for the comfort of the wounded. During the first year of the war a great amount of this work was devoted to the French. In the earlier months, especially, more was done for the French than for the British, as our new armies were not yet in the field, and the heroic efforts of France in beating back the invader and in holding her vast battle-front, with all the suffering it had cost her, demanded and received our ardent sympathies. All day in the depots there were women making sleeveless vests and bandages from French patterns; and at night numbers of women and girls, tired with a long office day, would come to spend their evenings in these labours of love. What more touching proof, to Frenchmen and Frenchwomen, of the feeling that France inspired? In one case at least, that of the Belgravia Supply Depot, the foundress was enabled to journey to France and visit many hospitals, in order to find out their individual needs; and this depot alone has sent supplies to over two hundred and fifty hospitals.

With the rapid and huge growth of our own armies, the ever-augmented number of fresh hospitals, and the ever mounting totals of sick and wounded, the supply depots – themselves continually expanding and increasing in number – became, naturally, more and more absorbed in the effort of providing for our own troops. But they have by no means ceased to send consignments to the French hospitals.

The Hospital Supply Depots (as also the Work Parties and Regimental Associations) worked, during the first year of the war, quite independently of each other. They worked independently also of the Red Cross Society, which strictly abstains, according to the Geneva Convention, from aiding any but the actually wounded soldiers. Hence much overlapping and a good deal of waste. Therefore in September 1915, the Army Council, determined to make all this voluntary effort as effective as possible, created a new department, that of the Director-General of Voluntary Organisations. This department has co-ordinated all this vast and widespread effort, organising it under officially recognised County, Borough, and District Associations. All work is done on requisitions sent out from the central office of the department. The gifts which are set apart for

French hospitals are usually sent to France either through the *Comité Britannique* or through the French War Emergency Fund. This last is an important society, whose activities call for a particular description, and to which we shall come in a moment.

Besides all these voluntary organisations in the British Isles, there are one or two similar enterprises carried on by English people in France. Such is the Society *'Pour les Blessés,'* which works in the bastion close by the Porte Dauphine in Paris, and makes simple surgical appliances not usually supplied to hospitals, and increasingly difficult to procure in adequate quantities, for the French wounded. The war has brought extraordinary ingenuity to bear on the problems of adjustment and support for broken limbs, and *papier-mâché* splints are made to suit every case. This society was formed under the authority of the French Government, and the *Service de Santé* supplies workrooms, lighting, and heating. The workers are chiefly English ladies, and give their services. The demand for the appliances far exceeds the production; and it is hoped to extend and develop the society's activities.

Private enterprise has also undertaken the collection of gifts and money for the French wounded; for example, the 'Anglo-French Aid Depot' at Dieppe, organised and managed by an English lady, which since September 1914 has distributed comforts of all kinds to the various French hospitals in the district. This depot also arranges to meet trains and help mothers and children who are travelling alone.

And again, there is a fund, promoted and administered by the wife of the Commandant of the B.R.C.S. convoys with the French armies, while working in a French hospital at Montreuil.

At the beginning of 1916 were started '*Ateliers pour Fabrication et Fourniture aux Hôpitaux de Guerre*,' which have done admirable work. These ateliers have been organised by a Scottish lady. She opened her first *ouvroir* at Mentone, where willing workers were found during the winter, and at Aix-les-Bains in the summer. Later, a workshop was started at Nice, and in the winter of 1917 a branch was opened at Marseilles solely for the making of light *papier-mâché* splints (invented by an Englishwoman), for which the ateliers have been specially noted. *Pilons* for the amputated, of a model invented by a Danish surgeon, are another appliance in which the ateliers have specialised.

This is perhaps the fittest place in which to say a word of the gifts to the French wounded from the British dominions.

Large supplies have been issued to each of the French Red Cross Societies by the Canadian Red Cross; and it has supplied some three hundred French hospitals direct. About five thousand cases of supplies are distributed from these stores every month. The French Government has done everything in its power to assist; it has built five large store-houses for the Canadian Red Cross and placed lorries at its disposal for distributing supplies, either to the stations of Paris, or directly to the hospitals. Canada has two hospitals in France for the French, and has given great gifts in cash.

Nowhere in the Empire has the name of France evoked more fervent feeling than in Australasia. Vast quantities of stores have been sent to the French hospitals (the clothing and comforts being noticeably the very best of their kind), and public collections have been an occasion, not of perfunctory giving, but of abounding and heart-prompted generosity. Complete figures are not available; but the collections made in Australasia for French War Relief Work to the end of 1917 cannot fall far short of £500,000. The Ligue Franco-Australienne, founded in December 1914, has given funds and sent a vast amount of clothing for wounded and active soldiers, *rapatriés*, widows, and orphans.

The New Zealand Hospital for Rapatriés and the unit of trained nurses sent by the Australian Red Cross will both be mentioned later on. But one may add here, in evidence of the eager efforts of Australasia to help, that many Australasians rejected for active service have joined the British Ambulance Convoys.

The South African Hospital at Cannes will be described in its place; and South Africa has also contributed gifts of money.

India and Ceylon, Singapore, Trinidad, Mauritius, Newfoundland, Malta, Gibraltar, all have collected sums and sent them to the French Red Cross for the relief of France's wounded.

And now we come to the French War (originally French Wounded) Emergency Fund.

At 44 Lowndes Square, in London – a house provided free for the purpose by the landlord – the fund has its headquarters. The house is no mere office for clerical business; it is the scene of strenuous labour, where ladies who are voluntary workers, unpack, sort, and pack again, the endless stores destined for hospitals in France. This is no light occupation. The bales which are to be despatched contain things like boots, deck-chairs, splints, crutches, games, as well as clothes and gauze and lint and drugs; operating-tables have occasionally to be sent, and now and then an X-Ray apparatus. And to pack neatly and well in square bales sewn up in sacking is an art requiring both skill and patience, not to speak of endurance. Also, after a time, it is not exciting. But here are cheerful givers of their time and toil, knowing what a joyful welcome each bale will have at the end of its long journey.

And let us not forget to record the generous act of the Pantechnicon Company, famous storers of furniture, who give to the Fund, three days a week, the use of vans and horses, and also storage free.

In one of the rooms at Lowndes Square you may see a large map of France marked out into '*régions*' and showing all those where the fund is active. There are now but few parts of the country where the military hospitals have not been served by the fund: its ubiquitous activity is astonishing.

It should first be explained that the fund concentrates its energies on the Military Hospitals of France, as distinguished from the Red Cross Hospitals. Since there are 4,307 military hospitals, there is plenty of scope even for the abounding energies of which the fund is mistress. Yet up to the end of 1917 no less than about 3,000 of these were supplied with needed stores, and nearly double that number of appeals were answered.

In London large purchases of hospital necessaries are made. Like the stores which come in from the provincial centres, they are made up into bales and forwarded across the Channel, direct to the hospitals requiring them.

In Paris, at the Porte Dauphine, close by the entrance into the Bois de Boulogne, is the fund's Paris entrepôt.

The stores are housed in two *baraques* – clean and roomy wooden warehouses among a row of others devoted to like purposes. Here all the various articles sent over from England are numbered and arranged in their proper places on the shelves, with an admirable neatness. There have been occasions when a sudden crisis made demands too urgent for London to supply in time, and the Paris warehouse was then able, by clearing out all its stock in a day and despatching it, to fulfil the need and superbly vindicate the title of the fund.

But how is it possible to know what all the military hospitals in France are in need of?

Do not imagine a promiscuous plumping of big bales of what shops call 'assorted articles' – a miscellaneous selection of things presumed to be of use – on unknown recipients. The method is as simple as it is efficacious. All that is needed is the constant service of a group of ladies, giving their whole time and energy to the unpaid work, and scattered about the provinces of France, with a supply of motor cars for their use. Need it be said that these indispensables are forthcoming?

The ladies in question, chosen for their knowledge of the French language and French ways, and for other winning attributes, have each a headquarters in some town at a central point of the region which they serve. And, driving cars put at the disposal of the fund, each of these delegates visits all the hospitals in her region, interviews the *Médecin-chef*, the heads of the *Pharmacie*, and the *Lingerie*, and talks to the nurses; and she is thus able not only to bring away a precise list of what each hospital requires, but to form an independent opinion of its merits as well as its needs.

The lists of requirements thus sent in are submitted to a

special committee at Lowndes Square; and if the committee is satisfied that the need is real and urgent, precisely those things are packed and despatched forthwith.

If you have ever seen the face, or shared the feelings, of a matron presiding over the unpacking of a Red Cross bale, which bulges with splendid promise of so badly needed bandages (let us say), but finally discloses through the ripped sacking and waterproof paper nothing but pyjamas after pyjamas (of which the hospital chances to have more than enough already), you will understand the beautiful satisfactoriness of the French War Emergency Fund's method. There is no waste, no overlapping.

And the workers themselves feel, I doubt not, well repaid for all they give by the knowledge of the reality of the help and the sincerity of the appreciation with which it is welcomed. Let us quote some sentences here and there from the letters received at Lowndes Square in a single week of last year, because these will say more than any eloquence.

Note that practically every letter has a word for what one of them calls the *'emballages si habilement confectionnés.'*

From a French Hospital Ship plying between Salonika and Toulon:

I cannot tell you how grateful I am for such a splendid stock of clothing, etc. How I longed for such a stock on my last voyage, for while in dock at Malta we had about four hundred survivors from the French troopship Santoy brought on board in a drenched and miserable condition, some of them badly wounded, having been crushed between the boat and the rafts as the ship was sinking. Naturally, most of them had lost all they had, so you may imagine what a comfort dry warm clothing would have been to us. Not even a comb saved among the officers, and my own had to go the round! Many, many thanks to you and the Society for such a splendid gift.

From Toulouse:

All the articles sent proved of the greatest value to our dear patients; you have done us an immense service, for our linen left something to be desired... Our patients thank you for all your generous gifts – linen, bed-tables, mattresses, blankets, and games.

From Marseilles:

The drugs are all the more welcome since they are now so costly in France.

From another Hospital at Toulouse:

All has arrived complete and in excellent condition. You can hardly imagine what a help it will be. Many of the things are out of our reach, and yet so useful : the rubber articles, the woollen things, etc

From St-Rémy de Provence:

If your country had ever to suffer what ours is suffering now, the hearts of Frenchmen would remember and do more than their utmost to return their generous and gallant brothers-in-arms all the kindness they receive from them today.

From l'Isle:

Your superb package has just arrived... We can use everything, even to the wrappings... Thanks, a thousand thanks, to have combined the useful and the agreeable in what you have sent. Our dear sons of France will love the people of Britain, already so much esteemed, all the more... And we, good Frenchwomen, share their enthusiasm. The scarcity and dearness of everything make us appreciate the gift the more keenly...

From Alais:

Each thing unpacked gave us an extreme pleasure. Much was lacking here... particularly the indoor clothes, for we had nothing left for our sick and wounded, but old waistcoats and trousers mended to excess... We shall remember your visit like that of one sent by God.

From Cavaillon:

What was our admiration, our surprise, our joy on undoing the bales. Nothing has been forgotten.

From Antibes:

Thanks to your kindness, some of our soldiers are now able gladly to stretch themselves on a *chaise longue* in the sun, and others to sit up more comfortably in bed, to write and play games.

From Marseilles:

Everything will be most useful, for the long duration of the war has greatly diminished and worn down our first year's stock.

From Prives:

What a solace, what an encouragement, to know that far from us generous hearts are working devotedly to alleviate the sufferings of the soldiers of France.

If you remember that these lines are extracted merely from some of one week's letters of acknowledgment, you will have an inkling of the extent and the beneficence of the work of this society during the three years and more of its activity.

When the Chairman of the Executive Committee and

the Secretary showed me the various rooms at Lowndes Square, and when I contemplated the piles of warm clothing, the crutches, the sticks, the chairs, the games, the little comforts, all arranged in order, my mind carried me away to distant hospitals in France: I saw the arrival, the un-packing; the folded empty clothes filled themselves with comforted limbs; I saw the pleasure in the eyes of wounded men getting up for the first time; I heard the laughter and jokes of their comrades, the talk between nurses and patients, as the things from England are shown and discussed and admired; the luxurious sinking-back into a new chair, the trying of a new air-cushion...

And how did this fund come into existence? It was an English lady who, with one or two friends first conceived the project of collecting medical stores and comforts and sending them to France. Once determined on, friends rallied to the idea as an effective means of proving this country's admiration for the French soldier.

This was in October 1914, when, as we have seen, the tremendous force and rush of the German onslaught on France had beggared at the outset all anticipations of hospital needs – just as the estimate of guns and munitions was also to prove so tragically inadequate.

The seizure of the chief industrial districts of France had intensified those needs; and inevitably they were increasing every day. Even the superb effort made by the French Government and nation to provide the *Service de Santé* with the means to care for the wounded, while all the national forces were taxed to repulse the enemy's invasion, proved quite insufficient to equip all the hospitals which had been hastily created. Indeed that would have needed years of previous preparation and organisation on a scale hitherto undreamed of.

Hence the project was of the utmost practical value. Willing helpers were not wanting. The work grew apace. London headquarters were found in Lowndes Square. The French Government granted free entry into the ports and free carriage on the railways for the supplies sent over by the Fund, and provided the warehouses in Paris at the Porte Dauphine.

With time, the character of the work has somewhat changed, and at the same time greatly extended. Originally the fund was intended to meet the great emergency of the German invasion. No such overpowering emergency has arisen since; but the long lines held by the French armies, the gigantic strain and burden thrown on them during the two years in which they bore all the brunt of the fighting on the Western front, the vast number of refugees which France has on her hands, besides the wounded and sick: all this has made the help of the French War Emergency Fund very acceptable to the Military Hospitals, which are not as a rule supplied by the French Red Cross. The French Red Cross has some seventeen hundred hospitals of its own to serve; and the fund has therefore decided to devote itself exclusively to the Military Hospitals.

For though these hospitals are equipped with what is absolutely necessary, and the shortages of 1914 have been made good, it can readily be imagined that there is endless scope for supplementing this with wheeled chairs, cushions, hot-water bottles, extra garments, invalid foods, and other comforts, of which no hospital probably ever gets quite as much as it would like.

Among these 'extras' is a mechanical bed, devised for the Fund, that can be adapted to various shapes: for carrying as well as for sitting or reclining.

In the course of rather more than a year some half-million garments and a quarter of a million bandages were distributed, among countless other things; and since then the amounts have greatly increased.

THE STORY OF THE HOSPITALS

1914

Visitors to Nice who take the tram or – rarely energetic – walk to Monte Carlo, along the road which climbs the hills and curves above the blue bays of the Mediterranean, will have passed a white building standing a little back from the road in a steep garden on the wooded face of Mont Boron.

This is the Queen Victoria Memorial Hospital. It was founded in 1906, and intended for such necessitous British or American visitors to the Riviera as were in need of hospital treatment.

When war broke out, the number of regular patients being few, and likely to grow greatly less, it was at once decided, on the 3rd of August 1914, to offer the hospital to the French Government for the use of the French wounded. The offer was gratefully accepted. The matron and assistant-matron were sent out, with other nurses, as quickly as possible; and in a short time the hospital began to take in sick and wounded from the French armies. Till November 1917 this was an *Hôpital Bénévole*, but in that month it was taken over by the French military authorities, the English staff remaining. This was, of course, an exceptional case. Practically all the hospitals we are to speak of were improvised for the needs of the war. And in these first months it was indeed a case of improvisation.

Each of us, I suppose, in looking back to those early days of a now irrevocably altered world, has in his memory some pictures more distinct than others, or remembers some moment that brought home to him with peculiar vividness the tremendousness of the events taking place with such fearful rapidity within what used to be but a few hours' journey from these shores.

Nothing of those memories comes back to the writer with a sharper shock than the sight, one August afternoon when he came out from his work into the streets, of an orange placard with the legend in great capitals – FALL OF NAMUR. So much had been staked upon the holding of that famous fortress. It was the pivot of the Allies' defending tactics. And it was gone, like a child's sandcastle in a rising tide! Could we have been there, we might have seen a group of English nurses – they were the only professional nurses in the place – tending the wounded, French and Belgian soldiers, women and children also, in a convent building. When they looked from their convent window, shaken every moment by the shocks of explosion, they could see columns of infantry and batteries of artillery clattering past with all the signs of hurry and confused retreat. A tragic mistake had been made. The huge German siege guns had been allowed to approach too near under cover of the summer mists; and the pounding to pieces of the forts, from a distance at which the Belgian guns could not answer, was a mere matter of time. And no long time either! Yet, so secure had the defenders felt themselves, that no plans for an orderly retreat had been made.

The English nurses remained with their wounded.

This record is not strictly concerned with the hospital and ambulance work done in Belgium. But at Namur there were French troops as well as Belgians, and here therefore our story begins.

It was on the 16th of August that this hospital unit of eight trained London nurses, with a surgeon from Guy's

– known as the Millicent Sutherland Ambulance – arrived at Namur. Just six hours after their arrival communications were cut. A hospital was installed in the Couvent des Sœurs de Notre Dame. Beds were prepared for the wounded in the large school of the convent, and the nuns undertook the cooking. All the beds were filled on the first day of the bombardment. Women and children were wounded by the bursting shells, and these had to be tended too.

The bombardment lasted three days. Then the Germans entered the town.

The English nurses were ordered to Maubeuge. But Maubeuge, when they reached it, was already in German hands, and there was no work for them to do. They were given passports to England, but, instead of arriving at Boulogne, found themselves in Brussels. Here they were ordered into Germany; but owing to the good offices of the American Minister, they succeeded in escaping to Holland, and thence home. Unfortunately all or nearly all of their medical and surgical supplies were lost on the journey.

Meanwhile much was doing, and feverish preparations were being made in England. During the Great Retreat of the Allies, when all was in suspense, more than one party of doctors and nurses was held up either in England or in French ports. But in the first fortnight of September the battle of the Marne was fought and won, and a new feeling was in the air.

Already an English hospital had been opened in the Paris. Hôtel Majestic in Paris, with some hundred beds, and a highly efficient staff. This was the first fruits of the enterprise of an English doctor, who on the eve of England's declaration of war had decided, should war break out, that he would devote himself to the organisation of hospitals for the wounded in France. Early in August he was in Paris, making plans in consultation with the French Red Cross, and returning to London got together his first unit, finally installed in the Majestic. Those were nightmare times. Here was a country suddenly called to fight for its life and to care for its wounded at the same time, when all ordinary conditions were dislocated, the traffic on the railways deranged and congested, accommodation of every kind inadequate to the fearful pressure of the moment, the resources of the medical service strained beyond all conception. Men would often be nine days in the train before proper surgical help could be given them. French, English, Belgian, and German wounded were brought indiscriminately to the Majestic; and the head surgeon would frequently operate on five or six cases during the night after twenty operations in the day. On one day, the founder of the hospital came upon nearly two hundred badly wounded men, lying for the moment with no medical service near. He brought as many as could be spared from the staff of the Majestic; for three days and a half continuously they worked to save these men; many they brought at last to Paris on barges. But by December Paris was fully provided with hospitals, and it was thought desirable to set to work elsewhere. The Majestic was therefore closed in January 1915. Returning to England during the second week of September, the founder of the enterprise collected in a few days a complete unit and full equipment for a large surgical hospital, which left London on 29th September, and was soon installed at Limoges, in the Musée Ceramique. At the beginning of 1915 this hospital was taken over by the Wounded Allies Relief Committee.

While passing through Dieppe with this unit, the doctor

saw that help was urgently needed in that town, and in answer to his urgent message a unit was brought over which eventually settled at Yvetot. Later, the same enterprise established an English hospital at Nevers. But these hospitals will be dealt with in their turn. Meanwhile let us return to Paris.

By the 12th of that September month, two complete hospital units, entirely composed of women, had left for France. They were under the charge of two eminent women surgeons. Part of the sumptuous Claridge's Hotel in the Avenue des Champs-Élysées was transformed into a hospital, the ground floor making lofty wards, full of air and sun.

The wounded, brought from as near the front as the motor ambulances were allowed to go, arrived often in a terrible condition. Tetanus and gangrene had appeared. On one day one of the women surgeons operated for seven hours at a stretch.

It is pleasing to record what a daily eye-witness said at the time:

> What the doctors won't tell you is their own admirable skill and devotion. The most awful and impossible-looking work is done by them as simply and quietly as if they were taking tea. There is something sublime to me in seeing such women, who will not even admit that they are doing anything out of the common. Everything is in order and ready to hand, and they go about their duties, just as if they were merely keeping house.

This is the testimony of a Frenchman, a wealthy stock-broker, who kept the door of the hospital-hotel. He had put his cashiers and clerks to sweep and scrub the floors;

but all on full pay.

Chiefly owing to the difficulty of finding fuel during the winter, the hospital was given up in January 1915, and the surgeons returned to take charge of the great Military Hospital in Endell Street, where none but women are on duty. On the 26th of September a hospital was opened by the Church Army in Normandy. The building, a school in the Rue de Bayeux, was lent by the municipal authorities. It contained a hundred beds. All the staff were British. The hospital was fully equipped with the most modern appliances and instruments; it had an X-Ray installation, and was entirely independent of outside help. Practically all the cases sent to the Church Army War Hospital were very serious surgical cases, and such patients naturally had to be kept for long periods. In April 1916, the hospital was closed down.

Many of the hospitals we are concerned in are installed in French châteaux.

An American lady, who owns a château at Longueil-Annel, north of Compiègne, in the department of the Oise, converted it into a small hospital at the beginning of the war. The German invasion swept through, and for a short time it was evacuated, but reopened on 27th September. A staff of doctors, nurses, and orderlies was procured through the British Red Cross Society; and an *ouvroir* was opened in rooms lent by the Hôtel Crillon, where stores and clothing are kept and distributed to convalescent soldiers, many of whom come from the invaded districts and lack for everything. In the early days the Annel Hospital was also able to help others in the neighbourhood.

Another château, which was converted to hospital use early in this September, was the old Château of St-Malo in Brittany. At St-Malo there is, of course, an English colony. And in the days after the Marne, when trainloads of the wounded were arriving in all the western towns, several members of the colony offered their services and aided in looking after the wants of the wounded. Over six hundred arrived on 17th September, and the hospitals were overflowing. At this juncture an offer arrived from a Red Cross Hospital at Bournemouth to send over a staff of trained nurses and doctors. An arrangement to install these in the Hôtel Franklin, which had just been turned into a hospital, fell through; but when the party landed from the boat on the evening of 22nd September, they found that part of the old Château of St-Malo had been placed at their disposal.

The château is a mediæval fortress with great stone ramparts, donjon towers and walls of formidable thickness; and the barracks within were not the most promising of buildings. There was no gas, no electricity, and water was laid on only on the ground floor. A regiment had only just left the barracks; the rooms were dirty; only three of them had been whitewashed and made ready for patients. But all set to work with a will, and soon had the place transformed.

All that the rooms contained of furniture was four tables and a few benches: so there was a busy day's buying of basins and pails, of kettles and brooms, and all the various utensils required in a hospital; while big bales of sheets and shirts, and lint and gauze, brought over from Bournemouth, were hastily unpacked, just in time for the arrival of the first wounded.

The English resident who has taken a chief part in establishing and maintaining the hospital at St-Malo had guaranteed, with a friend, the necessary sum for installing electric light and laying on a supply of water on every floor. But these things could not be accomplished in a day. In the meantime, dressings after nightfall had to be done by candle-light, and the water brought up from the kitchen to the wards and to the operating theatre on the second floor. Mistakes sometimes occurred, and a nurse would find herself pouring out cider for the surgeon to wash in. The rats of the old castle also came out to inspect the English invaders of their ancient home.

These are small details, but they help one perhaps to picture better the kind of difficulties that had to be overcome in most of the improvised hospitals of which we have to speak. Those who went out in those early days and took part in the vigorous transformations will never forget their effort and their victory over a hundred obstacles. What an elation the sense of serving a great cause gave to the toil, and what a new world of romance, if also of tragedy, they seemed to have entered!

After a few months' hard work in the château – cases of tetanus at that time were frequent, and the anti-tetanus serum was only to be procured with the greatest difficulty and at high cost – the hospital was required to move its quarters. The château was to be used once more as a barracks; and the hospital was transferred to the Hôtel des Grèves in St-Malo.

Another English hospital for the French had been established in St-Malo since 14th October. It was organised by the Order of St. John of Jerusalem, and originated in the following way.

About the middle of September, a French Médecin-Major called on an English Colonel, a resident of St-Malo. The Médecin-Major had been ordered to organise hospitals at St-Malo; but he had no instruments, drugs, dressings, etc., he was even without cotton-wool. Having heard that the Colonel was crossing to England, he asked him to procure and bring over whatever he could in the way of instruments and stores. During the last week of September, the Colonel returned from England with the stores which he had purchased, and not only with these, but with an offer from the late head of the Order of St. John to staff a hospital at St-Malo. The day after his return, the Colonel and his wife, with the Médecin-Major, inspected a girls' school called Moka – a building requisitioned by the French Government – and it was at once passed as suitable for a hospital.

Early in October the representative of the Order of St. John arrived, and it was arranged with the French authorities that the Hôtel Bristol at Paramé, close to St-Malo, should also be made into a hospital. On the 20th of the month, Moka having been put in order, the hospital staff arrived from England. The same day the first wounded arrived, and thenceforward the hospital was nearly always full.

The Moka was now known as *Hôpital Complémentaire* No. 62, the Bristol as *Hôpital Complémentaire* No. 94.

The Moka building was in itself excellently adapted for a hospital; the rooms were airy and well-lighted. Unfortunately the drainage system of St-Malo was being relaid at the time when war broke out, and the hotel had not been connected up either with the sewers or with the water. These conditions did not make for health. There were cases of typhoid and diphtheria; wounds refused to heal; the staff got bad throats; and in January 1915, the doctor in charge procured permission to transfer the hospital to the Hôtel

Bristol at Paramé.

The Bristol had been also converted into a hospital by the Order of St. John, and was opened a few days after the Moka. It was used for medical cases only till January 1915, when the original staff were recalled, and the Moka staff took their place.

It was no light job to move between eighty and a hundred patients in a single ambulance, as well as all the instruments, appliances, beds and bedding, stores and all the belongings of the staff, from the one hospital to the other; but it was done without any patient being out of bed for more than half an hour or missing a hot meal. This motor ambulance was the only one in the town, and was used freely by all the hospitals of St-Malo.

The Bristol Hotel, built on a rock above the sea-waves, had modern conveniences, a bath and hot water supply, and balconies facing the sea. There were 210 beds, most of which were always full. But the numbers became less, and the cases less serious, as the pressure of the first overwhelming urgency relaxed and the French *Service de Santé* got things into smoother going. It was therefore decided in April by the Order of St. John that the staff should be recalled. The hospital was handed over to the French. The instruments, bandages, etc., and also the X-Ray apparatus were handed over to them at the same time. There was only one other X-Ray installation in the town, with its twenty hospitals; so this was an appreciated boon.

Attached to these hospitals was a bacteriological laboratory, which was intended to serve not only the two St. John's hospitals, but the entire district. The doctor in charge of this laboratory was, in February, appointed official bacteriologist to the 10th Military Region; St-Malo, Dinan, and

Dinard being the centres of distribution. The laboratory did excellent work, especially in combating the spread of cerebro-spinal meningitis.

In connection with these hospitals, it should be recorded that a unit of seven surgeons and fifty nurses arrived at St-Malo from England on 1st November 1914, on the understanding that their services were needed by the *Service de Santé* at Rennes. Those members of this 'Rennes Unit' who remained in Brittany were distributed among various French hospitals in the district, some of which had English doctors or nurses from other sources. At the Hôtel des Terrasses, Dinard (*Hôpital Complémentaire* No. 52); the Hôtel d'Angleterre and Hôtel Longchamp at St-Lunaire (*Hôpital Complémentaire* No. 46); at a convent at Tréguier on the north coast (*Hôpital Complémentaire* No. 74); at Lannion (*Hôpital Temporaire* No. 20); and again at Dinard ('Canadian Hospital'), there were English workers forming part of the staff.

A party of surgeons, nurses, and others, all voluntary workers, went out in October 1914, and under the *Union des Femmes de France* opened a hospital of 107 beds at Fort Mahon in the department of the Somme. Coming under the control of the British Committee of the French Red Cross, this unit was enlarged by the addition, a few months later, by way of an annexe, of an evacuation hospital of thirty beds at Château de Boismont le Comte. A further addition to the formation was a Field Ambulance Corps of four ambulances. This unit worked on the Arras-Bethune front.

In this same October, the Millicent Sutherland Ambulance, Dunkirk. whose adventures in Belgium have already been recorded, resumed its activity. The lady who founded and directed the unit took over to Dunkirk a small convoy which did good work, already described in the chapter on the Convoys.

But if the ambulances were needed, there was equal need in this Dunkirk region of a hospital. At the request of the French, a hospital of ninety beds for 'Grands Blessés' was started at Malo-les-Bains, a little bathing-place near Dunkirk. The convoy also had its headquarters here. But in June 1915, repeated bombardments of Dunkirk made the place too dangerous, and the hospital was removed to tents at Bourbourg, a small town twelve miles to the south. In the autumn a return was made to Malo, but new dispositions of the armies had been made; the unit was asked to transfer its services to the British, and it has worked for the British Army at Calais ever since. The Directress had won the *Médaille des Épidemies*.

Another hospital of forty beds was established at Malo-les-Bains, in the Villa Belle Plage, by another English lady in November; and this was closed altogether in May 1915, again owing to the bombardments of Dunkirk.

Meanwhile, at Dieppe a hospital had been founded by an English doctor and his friends, in the buildings of the Hôtel de l'Alliance. The first patients were received on 10th October. But the accommodation was far too limited for the needs of the hour. The Commandant of the Third Division at Rouen offered the use of part of a large seminary building at Yvetot, on the main line between Rouen and Le Havre, the remainder of which was already occupied by a French Red Cross hospital; and the offer was accepted. The building was admirably adapted to its new uses. The dormitories formed spacious wards for the patients; the teachers' rooms, all on one corridor, housed the staff. A pavilion in the centre of the grounds made excellent offices for the administration. But the building had been disused for some years; it was in bad repair; and, as at St-Malo, it was necessary, besides cleaning and adapting the rooms, to provide heating, baths, and proper sanitary arrangements. Water, gas, and electric light were laid on throughout the hospital. All this meant large expense, and owing to lack of labour the alterations took some time to carry out.

Early in January 1915 the first ward was completed and the first wounded received. Two hundred and sixty-five beds were finally installed, and space left for fifty more. The original hospital at Dieppe was still maintained for a time.

A Convalescent Home was also established at the same time at Veules-les-Roses, a little place by the sea, twenty miles away, of which some few English people have pleas-ant holiday memories before the war.

To handle and control the financial and administrative side of the work, it was decided to form a committee, and out of this committee there arose a Benevolent Society which took the name of the Allies Hospital Benevolent Society, registered on 8th March 1915.

A particular feature of the Yvetot Hospital is the number of beds maintained by the heads and employees of large business firms in England, through small subscriptions. American help, in this as in other hospitals, has also been a strong support, and for several months Americans formed about a third of the staff. In August 1915 this contingent left to take up the work of a hospital at St-Valery-en-Caux.

A hospital, which was discontinued in the earlier part of 1915, was started in the first week of November 1914 by a lady well known for her hospital services the Balkan War. She was taken prisoner in Belgium with her husband in the first days of the war, and, having narrowly escaped being put to death by the Germans, organised a hospital for the Belgians at Antwerp. When that city was bombarded, the wounded were rescued, though the hospital material had perforce to be abandoned. She then brought her unit back to London, and shortly after established a hospital near Cherbourg, in the Château de Tourlaville.

Here again there was infinitely much to do before the building could be made ready for hospital use. The château was rebuilt in the time of Henri IV. With its old stone walls partly clothed in ivy, and projecting towers, square or octagonal, reflected in a lake and surrounded by trees, it has a peaceful beauty of aspect, though the history of its past is written in violent deeds and bloodshed. But it was built in an age which preferred dark staircases to spacious windows; and at the utmost it could only house seventy-five beds. Such a building is not ideal for a hospital. At the same time, from talks with French soldiers, one may gather that some at least of them get a certain pleasure from being nursed in an old château. It amuses their minds perhaps to be in a place that has a savour of history and romance about it; there is a mental background, however vague, which is a kind of repose and satisfaction to wandering thoughts and fancies, and which is certainly lacking to the finest of modern hospitals. But this, no doubt, is deplorable heresy.

With the exception of the treasurer and some of the chauffeurs, all of the staff at Tourlaville were women. And, as we shall see in the case of the Scottish Women's Hospital at Royaumont, there was at first a good deal of misgiving among the French, who doubted whether women surgeons were really capable of a serious operation. However, a distinguished surgeon of the district came to visit the hospital; witnessed an operation, and recorded his emphatic opinion that at Tourlaville '*les chirurgiennes sont de valeur égale aux chirurgiens les meilleurs.*'

In the garden of the château a large marquee was set up with a boarded floor and with stoves to heat it. This was used as a recreation tent for convalescents. Bought with subscriptions from workers on a ranch in British Columbia, it was later to go to Serbia, and is now in the hands of the enemy. For in February 1915 the *Directrice* herself decided to go to Serbia, where there was a lamentable scarcity both of doctors and nurses. Typhus was raging there. One third of the Serbian doctors had died, either killed in the firing-line, or carried off by the epidemic. And less and less wounded were coming to Tourlaville. They came to Cherbourg by sea, and the sea passage was dangerous. The hospital continued under other direction for a short time; but the number of wounded continued to decrease, and the hospital was closed at the end of March 1915.

And now we return to Dunkirk, whence the wounded were transported by sea to Cherbourg, some, inevitably, dying on the way. The race for Calais and the coast, after the victory of the Marne, had brought the war suddenly into this region. The pressure was as overwhelming as it was unexpected; it was almost impossible to cope with the numbers of wounded during those tremendous struggles on the Yser, and the days of the first battle of Ypres. Some English efforts to help have been recorded; and now a Scottish lady, hearing of the urgent need, organised an ambulance with an English staff, and opened it at Malo-les-Bains in a villa on the sea lent by its French owner. An X-Ray installation, much needed, was brought out with the unit. The hospital was opened on 20th November, and until 1st June its seventy-five beds were practically always full. After the first gas attack in April on the Ypres salient, the wounded arrived in such numbers that they were laid on mattresses in the floors and vestibules, every bed being occupied. The hospital escaped damage in the bombardment of Dunkirk; but on June 1st it was closed for the time being, as no more wounded were arriving, and finally removed in November. Its work, however, had been so much appreciated that the foundress was asked to transfer it to Paris, which was done at the end. of 1915, and we shall describe its further activities in their place.

Before the end of 1914 both sides had settled down to the trench warfare, which was to continue so long. Conditions being now more or less stationary, it was possible to deal with Red Cross problems more deliberately, to reorganise much that had necessarily been in a fluid state while the armies were in movement, and to ensure a more methodical working.

As yet, however, the hospitals near the front were comparatively few. Consequently the wounded, even the seriously wounded, were being evacuated to hospitals which were often at great distances from the front, in the south, the south-west, and the west. We shall see how this condition of things gradually changed, and how the change affected some of our hospitals. A case in point is the history of the next unit of which we have to give an account.

This is the Ulster Volunteer Hospital.

The outbreak of war on the Continent found a section of the Ulster Volunteers, the North Tyrone section, with medical staff and equipment for two thousand men, all in readiness for the contingency of war in Ireland. How could this staff be used? An offer was made in the first instance to the British War Office – as was done in some other cases – but it came to nothing; and a proposal was then made to the French authorities through a Bordeaux lady. An invitation came speedily, asking the unit to go to Pau. The party sailed from Liverpool in October, reached Pau on the 12th, and found that the Villa Beaupré had been placed at their disposal. There were fifty beds: all too few, as it happened, for the ample staff sent out. But no sooner was the *Préfet* made aware of this superabundance of skilled energy than he asked to borrow from it for a hospital in the neighbourhood. Two orderlies and two probationers were lent to this French hospital, under two Sisters: one of these Sisters has been there ever since, and is reported to have done invaluable work.

At this time, as we have said, the wounded were coming as far south as Pau direct from near the front; even from places as far away as Dixmude. But gradually the hospitals nearer the front were reopened, and bad cases kept there till they were better able to support the long journey south. At the Villa Beaupré the number of beds had been increased to sixty, and later to eighty; but by the beginning of 1916 serious cases were becoming fewer and fewer, and the patients were practically all either in an early stage of convalescence, or men with slight wounds from the Champagne front. But light work is not to the mind of doctors and nurses. They crave for arduous days and nights; they hunger for difficulties and desperate cases; they want to be used to the last of their strength and experience; not to fulfil a prescribed duty only, but to give all they can, and all they know.

In February the first crash of the tremendous German assaults on Verdun was echoing over Europe. And in the spring of 1916, the hospitals in the central regions of France were busy indeed. It was decided that the Ulster Volunteers should move to Lyons, but it was not till the end of April that the hospital was closed at Pau. The unit reached Lyons on the 2nd May, but much had to be changed and improvised in the building put at their disposal, and it was not till the beginning of June that patients began to be received. The building was a technical school, owned by a society, the '*Travail de la Femme et de la Jeune Fille*'; and it accommodates a hundred beds. It is not in Lyons itself, but in an outlying suburb on the south of the city.

December 1914 was a month which saw the establishment of several more hospitals, some of which are of special interest. Already, in November, a hospital staff, with three motor ambulances, was on its way to France from South Africa, and during the winter was being installed in a large hotel at Cannes; but as it was not actually ready for work till February, we will reserve our account of it for the moment.

Three hospitals which were opened in this December have since been closed. The *Hôpital Anglo-Français* at Le Tréport, on the coast between Dieppe and the mouth of the Somme, was founded by an English lady, and was housed in a golf hotel. It was opened on the first day of the month. The wounded came direct from the fighting line at Arras, Souchez, Neuville St-Vaast, and Notre Dame de Lorette – places now so familiar on our lips, since our own men have fought and fallen there. When our troops took over the line, the hospital was closed for French wounded on 10th June 1916, but it was reopened in July as a British Red Cross Hospital for British officers; as such it is still working.

Another hospital was established by an English lady in the Casino at Fécamp. It was called *Hôpital Anglais du Casino*, and opened on 6th December; the people of the town warmly welcomed the English staff. This was discontinued on 14th June 1916, when the French sent no more wounded in that direction.

At Nevers, in the very centre of France, was started a hospital which has been already mentioned in conjunction with two others, one in the Hôtel Majestic, Paris, and the other at Limoges. The Nevers hospital is on the outskirts of the town, with open fields about it: it was housed in some quite modern buildings which were erected as offices for the P.L.M. Railway Company. From the start, in December 1914, until its close in the autumn of 1917, the hospital was filled with patients. The number of beds, originally 110, was afterwards increased to 170. There being no accommodation for nurses in the hospital itself, they were lodged in neighbouring châlets.

It was in December 1914 also that a hospital known as the Anglo-Ethiopian Hospital was opened at Frévent in the Pas-de-Calais. His Majesty's Chargé d'Affaires in Abyssinia had offered a hospital to the French Government in September; it had been accepted; and, after some considerable difficulties in finding a suitable building and getting together the necessary staff and equipment had been overcome, it was installed in a hospice belonging to the town of Frévent, and began to receive patients. For some four months, while constant fighting was going on in the Arras region, the hospital's sixty-seven beds were occupied mostly by men with severe wounds, many of whom could not have travelled farther. But in the following April all privately conducted hospitals were moved from the zone in which

Frévent lies, to be replaced by military ambulances; and the Anglo-Ethiopian Hospital was transferred to St-Valery-sur-Somme, where the Casino had been allotted to it. Here also the cases were often serious, and the many patients remained for long periods. The wounded were fetched from Abbeville in the English cars attached to the hospital. In October 1915 the hospital was handed over as it stood, together with a sum of money to pay for the heating of the Casino during the winter, and for the maintenance of a French staff, to the *Service de Santé*. The head of the staff had obtained permission to take out a nursing unit to staff a French military hospital in the island of Tenedos, and left St-Valery on this new mission. The unit worked at Tenedos till the French left the island, when it was lent for an indefinite period to the Royal Naval Division, and worked partly at Tenedos, partly at Mudros and at Imbros.

It is to be recorded that the Anglo-Ethiopian Hospital was helped by a contribution from an Imperial Prince of Abyssinia in the shape of a gift of cattle, which were sold for a good sum.

Just before Christmas another hospital was opened in the Pas-de-Calais, at Berck-Plage, by the Glamorgan and Monmouthshire Hospital Committee. Berck had just been taken over as a hospital centre for one of the French armies, and a number of military hospitals were being improvised in the Casino, the hotels, and other large buildings that were available. The Hôtel de Russie was obtained for the Glamorgan and Monmouthshire Hospital – now known officially as *Hôpital Auxiliaire Anglais*, Annexe No. 44 – through the efforts of the lady who acted throughout as *Directrice*. It accommodated one hundred beds. There were no motor ambulances in Berck, except those belonging to this British hospital; and on its staff therefore fell the work of bringing the wounded away from the station, and distributing them among the various hospitals in the town. Not till May 1915 was there set on foot a system of regular convoys bringing the wounded down from the front by road. Most of the cases at the hospital were cases of severe wounds, involving a long stay. By July 1915 it had become apparent that the French Medical Service in Berck was thoroughly well established, and further assistance was not needed. The hospital was therefore closed, and the whole of its excellent equipment and stores of clothing was made over to the French military authorities.

From the same month of December dates the opening of the Scottish Women's Hospital at Royaumont.

The fateful 4th of August found the Women Suffragists of Scotland with a powerful organisation: and their first thought was how best to use its means to help the sufferers from the war. It was decided to staff and equip hospitals for foreign service, the prime mover being the late Dr. Elsie Inglis. A committee was formed, and an appeal issued; and money flowed in from all classes in the country.

It was through the good offices of the *Présidente* of the *Comité Britannique* that the Cistercian Abbey of Royau-mont was placed at the disposal of the Scottish Women's Hospitals Committee. It is on the skirts of the forest of Carnelle, in the valley of the Oise; seven miles from the railway at Chantilly, and twelve from Creil, the junction on the line from Calais to Paris. After sheltering for centuries more than one religious order in turn, the Abbey buildings had been put to industrial uses. But for ten years it had been abandoned, disused; and the immense rooms were littered with hay, timber, stone fragments from the destroyed church, and all manner of odds and ends and rubbish. All this had to be cleared away by the Scottish Women, with no male hands to help them, before the task of cleaning could be begun. They were then confronted by the absence of water, light, and heat. But nothing could daunt their intrepid spirits. Electric light, heating, sanitary arrangements were all rapidly installed, though there is no considerable town in the neighbourhood. The outfit and stores from Edinburgh arrived by railway at the distant station, and had to be transported by the chauffeuses to the Abbey, and there carried up flights of stairs to the floors for which the sets of bales were destined. With a fever of enthusiastic energy the whole staff – doctors, nurses, and orderlies – joined in the giant task of cleaning and preparing the vast collection of buildings. At last all was ready and in the nicest of order.

But where were the wounded?

We have seen already that there was a certain doubt existing in the French mind as to the competence of women surgeons and doctors. Could the wounded be trusted into their hands? The eager staff waited; but their newly arranged wards, the pride of their hearts, remained empty. At last a remonstrance addressed to the authorities evoked an inspection. Certificates of qualification were demanded; they were at once produced. The wards had been arranged on the upper floor. This was not approved: it was decided that the lower floor was the proper floor for them. More days of toil! But the labour was cheerfully surmounted, and the new wards made as perfect as the old.

Still the wounded delayed. At last six arrived, but they were sick, not wounded. And then came the change. The French discovered very soon the quality of the work of the

Scottish Women. Curiosity was provoked; visits were made by doctors in high places; admiration was spontaneous and cordial. It was not long before the French authorities were asking that the original eighty beds should be increased to two hundred. Later the number became three hundred, and finally four hundred. If there had been diffidence at first, it was amply made up for by the warmth of recognition when it was seen how admirably these women of Scotland could administrate, organise, operate and nurse. Recently the *Médaille des Épidémies* has been conferred on thirty members of the staff; and in September 1916 the President of the Republic himself journeyed to Royaumont to inspect the hospital and express his appreciation. One of the Royaumont wards has been equipped by Canada.

A few months after the opening of the hospital, the work done at Royaumont was so greatly esteemed that an invitation came to the committee from the French military authorities to establish another hospital at Troyes, the ancient capital of Champagne, on the Eastern Railway. The offer was accepted with pride, and no pains were spared to make this second hospital as perfect as was possible.

Not in Troyes itself, but about a mile from the town, the staff were housed in the Château de Chanteloup, which has old gardens and spacious grounds about it. The hospital itself was in tents. It was one of the first attempts to nurse the French wounded under canvas.

The unit was known as the Girton and Newnham Unit, since members of those famous women's colleges at Cambridge had contributed so large a sum towards its equipment. It was under the direction of Mrs. Harley, sister of Lord French, who had already worked at Royaumont.

But the unit had only been at work some months when an

order arrived from the French War Office to evacuate the hospital and proceed at once to Salonika with the French Expeditionary Force. The order was promptly obeyed. From Salonika the unit moved up-country to Guegvueli. But the Bulgarians and Germans were then advancing with formidable swiftness; and it was decided to retire to Salonika. There the hospital was extended to three hundred beds.

Here falls to be recorded the noble death of Mrs. Harley. She had given devoted service; she was to give her life also. In June 1915 she returned to England. In July of the following year she took charge of a flying column of motor ambulances attached to the Serbian Army in Macedonia. They were in camp at Ostrovo, and fetched the wounded from the front to the Scottish Women's Hospital at that place. This work among the mountains was dangerous and difficult, and Mrs. Harley's unit won especial praise both for its skill and its endurance. She was decorated by General Sarrail with the *Croix de Guerre*.

In December 1916 Mrs. Harley undertook the establishment and charge of an independent soup-kitchen and relief system for the civilian refugees at Monastir. On 7th March 1917, while seated at a window, she was wounded in the head by a shell which burst in the street, for the Bulgarians and Germans were bombarding the open town. She died almost immediately in the hospital to which she was taken.

1915

In the first month of 1915, two more hospitals were opened: one at Compiégne, and one at Arc-en-Barrois, while a third, already existing, at Limoges, was taken over into new control and enlarged.

Arc-en-Barrois – the Barrois is the old name of that district of Eastern France of which Bar-le-Duc is the centre – is a large village or little town lying in a pleasant valley among the rolling uplands and vast forests of the Haute Marne. It is about forty miles from the firing-line.

The *Hôpital Temporaire* at Arc is under the direction of a Worcestershire lady who had originally intended to take out a small party to nurse in a French hospital; but so many good workers joined the group that it soon grew into a complete unit of the St. John's Ambulance Association. The staff was approved by the Anglo-French Committee and the unit accepted by the French Government. The Duc de Penthièvre had offered his château at Arc to the Ministère de la Guerre, and here the hospital was finally installed.

The large rooms of the chateau made excellent wards on two floors: but there is no hot water laid on, no gas or electricity, no system of heating, and the same difficulties had to be overcome as in similar cases already described. All sorts of hospital furniture, such as the little tables which the patients like to have by their beds to keep their belongings on, as well as cupboards, fracture-beds, splints, etc., were made by amateur carpenters among the orderlies (all, in this case, English volunteers). An out-of-door ward, with a penthouse against the southern wall of the château, was also made, for the medicine of fresh air has been used as much as possible.

The château looks on a park, with streams running through it. No hospital is more fortunate in its surroundings; a matter of great moment for the wellbeing of the convalescent. This hospital has no beds. Shortly after it was opened, more room was required, and a Hospice standing on higher ground, on the outskirts of the little town, was taken over for the use of patients who were recovering, or who did not need an operation. This brought the total up to 180.

The Hospital of Arc served for a long time the Third Army, the army of the Argonne, where hard fighting was pretty continuous during 1915, while the Crown Prince was vainly endeavouring to break through and join up with the armies on his left. During the following year it was kept extremely busy by the tremendous battles of Verdun.

The entire staff at Arc-en-Barrois is English, with the exception of the French Administrateur and French 'Vaguemestre'; but local workers have given useful help.

Yet nearer to the front than Arc, and in fact only six or seven kilometres from the French front trenches, is another château, the Château Rimberlieu, some miles north of Compiègne, in which an Anglo-French hospital was installed by an English lady. Here again are spacious grounds and shady trees. The hospital contains some eighty beds; but in the spring of 1916, at the suggestion of the French authorities, an annexe was added – a large hut or *baraque* connected by a covered way with the main building, and containing another thirty beds, besides rooms for baths and for the dressing of wounds. At the Château Rimberlieu the staff was at the outset entirely British, but gradually changes have come about, and more recently the French element has predominated.

The hospital at Limoges, which was started in October 1914 was in this January taken over by the Wounded Allies Relief Committee. This society, formed at the beginning of the war, began by giving help to the Belgian wounded; it went on to aid both French and British hospitals in France with supplies and funds; and now, with the opening of the year 1915, it took over the hospital installed in the Musée Céramique at Limoges, which was no longer able to maintain itself for lack of funds. At the same time as the transfer, the number of beds was increased from 150 to 225.

In the next month, February, the Wounded Allies Relief Committee were invited to take over a hospital at Dieppe which was in the same case. This, the parent of the Yvetot Hospital, has already been described. It was decided to take over this hospital also. But as the hotel which housed it – the Hôtel de l'Alliance – could accommodate but sixty beds, and the expenses were high, it was eventually resolved to remove it to a larger building. The ampler quarters desired were found at Lyons, in the Lycée de St-Rambert; this is a big school-building on a wooded spur of the hills overlooking the Saône, with good air and a magnificent view. The removal was made in February of 1916.

This hospital has three hundred beds, and has also sheltered eighty homeless Serbian children. It lies on the other side of the city from the Ulster Hospital, already described, which also came to Lyons after being started elsewhere.

It has been mentioned that during this first winter a hospital unit from South Africa arrived in France, and was gradually installed at Cannes in the Hôtel Beau-Rivage. It had been organised in the first month of the war by members of the *Société Française du Cap*, and placed under the command of a distinguished South African French doctor, Lieutenant-Colonel in the S.A.M.C. The original accommodation in the hotel was for 150 patients, but the committee has since been asked to double the number. In February 1915 the hospital began active work.

How different were conditions here from those of the hospitals improvised in old châteaux, lacking every modern appliance! The Hôtel Beau-Rivage, built round a quadrangle roofed over from a central hall, is beautifully ventilated; its rooms and passages are commodious; above all, it enjoys the sea and the sun. From the sea it is separated only by its own garden, and it faces full south. The rays of the sun are used to help the surgeon, and with marvellous effect.

Besides the hotel, a large villa and garden adjoining it, placed at the disposal of the ambulance, has been maintained by the committee, and has housed numbers of officers, both French and Serbian, who, though discharged from hospital, were not sufficiently recovered to return to duty.

The admirably complete equipment of this hospital has enabled it to do considerable services not only for the wounded, but for the civil patients in Cannes. The laboratory and the X-Ray installation serve all the hospitals in the town.

Later on the ambulance put out an offshoot. This is a sanatorium, housed in the Villa Félicie, a villa with delightful gardens on the slope of the hills above Cannes. The villa was lent for the purpose by its English owners. Here are treated cases of early or threatened consumption; men suffering from chest and lung trouble which, if treated in an ordinary hospital, would develop into some form of tuberculosis.

A number of more hospitals in different parts of France were started in this spring of 1915. The first of these, known as the *Hôpital Wemyss*, was personally superintended by the lady who founded it, and the Château du Fayel, a magnificent house, was lent for the purpose by the French Duchess who owns it. There were many difficulties in the way of equipment and transport, but these were overcome, with the help of the French authorities, and work began in February. An offer had been made to maintain the hospital for a period of six months at least. It received wounded from Compiègne from February to October 1915, when, owing to the high expenditure involved, the *Directrice* reluctantly closed it.

On the 15th of February a hospital was opened at Neu-illy-sur-Seine by an English committee. Accommodation was found in a villa in the Boulevard Victor-Hugo, with an annexe connected with the house by a covered way, and a wooden pavilion in the garden. The villa had been a private sanatorium, so that it was well suited for its purpose. The number of beds, at first forty, were raised in March to fifty, and in August to seventy-five. The medical and nursing staff were British, with the exception of an American surgeon and a Swiss V.A.D. The English doctors were homoeopathic physicians who gave their services as their home practice permitted. The cases treated were chiefly surgical. Some well-known Paris surgeons helped by consultations. The hospital was closed in March 1916, as the proprietor of the building required it for the resumption of his sanatorium, and also the calls on doctors at home made it increasingly difficult for them to give their time to France.

In the same month a fully equipped hospital of fifty beds was presented to the French by the English lady who became its *Directrice* and by an English gentleman; and this was accepted as an annexe (Annexe Tangye) to the French *Hôpital Militaire* No. 35, at Paris-Plage, and installed in an hotel with sunny balconies. The nurses are English, the *Directrice* being *Infirmière Major*; the surgeons French. The cases treated have all been surgical; the nursing staff has won high appreciation from the French; and the relations between the French and English staff have been those of cordial understanding and goodwill.

At the beginning of March a hospital was opened at Dunkirk, which differs from the other hospitals of our record in being devoted not only to French but to British wounded. This is the Queen Alexandra Hospital, and is the most important of the hospitals set on foot and managed by the Friends' Ambulance Unit, whose convoy work has already been described.

The hospital is installed in wooden sheds, white-plastered, with garden plots about them. In the grounds are tents for infectious cases. The hospital has grown considerably, since it was first started. It now has two hundred beds, eighty for French soldiers, a like number for British soldiers, and forty for British sailors. The beds required by the French were originally under forty in number, but in the autumn of 1915 were increased to eighty. Structural alterations and additions were also made; equipment and fittings improved. Among other necessaries, a spacious dug-out was provided for use in case of air-raids; and, as we know, Dunkirk is liable to these attentions pretty constantly. In October 1915 the staff was augmented by a number of V.A.D. nurses. A dental surgeon has been given a room in the hospital, and is kept uncommonly busy.

A strange medley of races is to be found in this hospital of the Friends. Strolling about the grounds may be seen British sailors in their navy blue, and soldiers in khaki side by side with French infantrymen and Algerians and Fusiliers Marins with their red pompon on their caps, and not only these but Chinese and Egyptians and negroes from the West Indies. It is a hospital of good understanding and good fellowship.

Our next hospital has a special character, since it was planned for the exclusive service of the seriously wounded, '*les blessés qui peuvent mourir*,' and it was placed directly under the *Service de Santé* on the understanding that only fully trained nurses should be employed. It was therefore named the Urgency Cases Hospital for France. The project was that of the lady well known as Hon. Secretary of the National Union of Trained Nurses.

The unit left London on nth March 1915, and arrived at Bar-le-Duc on the 13th. A wing of the *Hôpital Central* in the town had been allotted to it. The first wounded arrived on the 23rd.

It was the only British unit in the Meuse, and attracted many visitors from the neighbourhood. Since it was soon recognised that it was not practicable for the unit to be placed in the first line, where really urgent cases were dealt with, the heads of the staff consulted together, and decided to specialise in some particular branch of surgery. The treatment of fractures was therefore chosen.

Six months were spent at Bar-le-Duc, where the hospital treated the wounded from the Argonne, and got all too well acquainted with the horrors of 'gas gangrene.' During the month of July, a formidable assault of the Germans in the Argonne forest nearly penetrated the line. The ambulances at the front could not cope with the incoming stream of wounded, and the hospital at Bar-le-Duc rendered a real service by fetching wounded from Les Islettes and St-Ménehould, and filling its wards to overflowing.

But a still more strenuous time was in store for the unit. In August 1915 the wing of the *Hôpital Central* which it occupied had to be taken over by the French; and a removal was made to Revigny, rather nearer the front. An empty château, called 'Faux Miroir,' was placed at the unit's disposal. It had proved its name, for it was the headquarters of the Crown Prince at the moment when the sanguine onrush of the Germans was turned into retreat.

The house, which stands in a park near the much-battered village of Revigny, would contain, it was found, the staff, but not the patients. For these, huts had to be built in the grounds. Water-pipes had to be laid on, the electric cable relaid, paths cut, drains cleaned. Yet in a fortnight of glorious effort all was ready. The number of beds was about one hundred, soon increased to one hundred and twenty.

Troubles with water-supply and electric currents, and, when the winter came, with leaking roofs and burst pipes, did not interfere with the work. And then in February came the great onslaught on Verdun.

On the morning of 13th February came an order to clear the hospital of wounded as quickly as possible. The order was carried out, only a few serious cases being retained. The great attack had not yet begun, but many signs of it had been seen and noted. On the 21st a fleet of aeroplanes twice bombarded Revigny, already so wrecked in the days of the retreat from the Marne. But it was not the buildings that was their target; it was the railway. They were driven off by gun-fire, having failed in their object. The same night another attempt was made to cut the line of communication to Verdun; this time by a Zeppelin. Members of the staff at Faux Miroir, who had already had the excitement of watching the attack and retreat of the aeroplanes, had gone up the hill after dark, to see what could be seen; the presage of events was in the air. Returning, they saw two long beams of light shoot out from earth to sky, then a third. And suddenly out of the darkness, trapped in the luminous beams, appeared a Zeppelin. In a moment guns began. The airship, distinct to the watchers below, started to crumple up towards one end; it sagged, then burst into flames, and plunged downwards slowly, trailing fire behind it. The Zeppelin was destroyed. And the two guns and the searchlights which had been its doom had been brought to Revigny that very day! A thrilling prelude this to the next six months of breathless work, while the gigantic attacks on Verdun hammered in vain at the fortress and the wounded arrived without ceasing. This was a happy time for the Faux Miroir staff; they were doing what they had come out to do. In July 1917 the hospital was handed over as it stood to the *Comité Britannique* of the French Red Cross, under whom it is still working.

No such excitements as those just recorded could be expected for the next unit on our record, *Hôpital Auxiliaire de l'Entente Cordiale* No. 222. For Mentone is far from the thunder of the guns, and lies out of reach of the enemy's aircraft; and though the Mediterranean is infested with U-boats, no spasm of shelling from an emerging submarine has disturbed its basking bay.

At the beginning of 1915, a former English resident of Mentone and his wife went to Mentone with the generous intention of starting a hospital there for the French wounded, but finding that the municipality of the town had expressed a desire to open a hospital for British officers and soldiers, in appreciation for all that English visitors had done for the place, they joined in an offer made to the British authorities. This came to nothing. An offer was then made to the *Association des Dames Françaises*, one of the three great Red Cross Societies, and in the result it was arranged that a hospital of four hundred beds should be installed in the building of the Hôtel Impérial, which was requisitioned by the French Government. This building was taken over for the purpose by the military *Service de Santé* free of rent, though with responsibility for dilapidations.

The hospital was opened under the auspices of the *Association des Dames Françaises* at the beginning of April. The original English donors paid for the whole outlay and maintenance of the hospital till mid-July, when an English Committee, formed for the purpose, began to support the work financially and undertook to collect subscriptions in England. The donors acted as Administrateur and *Directrice* respectively till, after a year of uninterrupted work, they felt obliged to retire. From April 1916 the English Committee took charge of the hospital.

This hospital, like the South African Hospital at Cannes, which has already been described, enjoys all the advantages and amenities of a modern hotel; but it is on a still larger scale, and being of more recent construction than the Hôtel Beau-Rivage, is still more luxurious in its arrangements. It goes without saying that there are lifts, electric lighting, central heating, bathrooms on every floor. Nothing, too, has been spared to perfect its equipment, so that the hospital has become the surgical centre for the Mentone district. It possesses an admirable pharmacy; a microbacteriological laboratory; a dark room for laryngology; a laundry with mechanical apparatus for washing and drying. On the ground floor is a room for aseptic operations which communicates with the sterilising room; and this in turn communicates with the radiography room, splendidly equipped by an Irish donor.

The hotel fronts full south. It stands at a certain elevation, with gardens sloping down to the sea, which it overlooks. As at Cannes, wonderful cures have been made by the help of the strong sun.

On the 20th of April a hospital was opened in the Gare Maritime, Cherbourg. The waiting-room for boat passengers, and rooms adjoining, were lent by the Cherbourg Chamber of Commerce; they accommodated sixty beds; and as the hospital is built out over the water, it could not have healthier air or more restorative surroundings. The Directress and nurses were English: the surgeons were also English, but an American surgeon was in charge for some months, and French doctors helped. For a short time in 1916 a Belgian Army officer was in charge. In 1916 the hospital was transferred to the Cherbourg Committee of the French Red Cross, the Director of which had done all in his power to help the hospital while it was maintained and managed by the English. The whole of the installation was handed over to that committee.

In May a hospital of thirty-five beds was opened at Ceret, in the *Pyrenées Orientales*, by an English lady, who was lent the house of a friend for the purpose. The delightful country and climate made it especially suitable for convalescents, and it was used mainly for wounded who were sent on from other hospitals in the Montpellier district; from places like Perpignan and Amalie-les-Bains. The hospital, known as *Hôpital Bénévole* No. 62 bis (Fondation Allhusen No. 1), did excellent service till it was closed on the 1st of February 1917. Meanwhile, the lady who had called it into being had started another hospital at Martouret, of which we will speak in its place.

On the 1st of May a hospital was opened at Gezaincourt, close to Doullens, just on the borders of the departments of Pas-de-Calais and Somme, and only about ten miles from the trenches. The building was a château, in a pleasant park, lent by its owner. It was supported by voluntary contributions from Ireland, and was known as the *Hôpital Irlandais*. Owing to its closeness to the front line, the cases received were of the worst and most dangerous wounds. It was closed in March 1916, owing to the British taking over the part of the line it served.

Many had hoped since the battle of the Marne that, with the advent of the summer, the Germans might be driven back from their strong positions in France and Flanders. And in May the coming of Italy into the war on the side of the Allies strengthened these hopes. Looking back, we are perhaps inclined to forget how sanguine we were, and how continually our eager expectations have been postponed. I think that few of those who founded the English hospitals we are describing had any anticipation that the war would last so long as it has. And when one considers the endless drain in ever new directions on the resources of English generosity, and the burden laid on those responsible for the continued maintenance – and in many cases the expansion – of these improvised hospitals, all the greater will be our appreciation of the fine tenacity which has been shown, and the splendid support which has been given by the people of Britain. This is a testimony to the strength of the feeling for France in this country. It was no transient enthusiasm. July 14th, the day of France's national festival, the day of the taking of the Bastille, was celebrated in London and the provinces, and collections made on behalf of the French Red Cross. A great sum was raised, to be surpassed in 1916, and again nearly doubled in the following year. But of France's Day and its collections we have already given some account.

The next hospital to be described has a special interest because, unlike the others, it is a field hospital. In July 1915 it was established at the little town of Rousbrugge in Belgium, and was attached to the French Army on that part of the front. The Englishwoman to whom the scheme was originally due had crossed to Dunkirk in February, the day the submarine blockade was declared by the Germans – and offered help to the French in their typhoid hospitals, which were at the time in need. She took with her two English nurses, and the three being drafted into different hospitals in the locality, she was able to help not only by actual nursing, but by providing hospital requisites and fittings. But the desirability of a field hospital, near the lines, which should be perfectly equipped, and so able to perform the most difficult operations without the delay of sending the wounded back to the base, presented itself more and more urgently. And before many months were over this idea reached its practical embodiment at Rousbrugge. The lady who had originated the scheme provided the huts, which were made on the spot, and the fittings, beds (about 160 in number), furniture, and surgical requisites, a large proportion of which were sent from England; she also provided the nursing staff, of which she was Directress. English subscribers liberally helped with gifts. The hospital was made over to the French Army, which supplied food, medical service, and medicines. From the outset the hospital has admirably fulfilled the functions it was intended to perform. It has moved two or three times; on one occasion because it was severely bombed, when a nurse and several patients were injured.

During the Somme campaign new work was taken up at

Bray-sur-Somme. The Field Hospital in Belgium continued its work, under the charge of an American nurse, since
awarded the *Médaille des Épidémies*, while the Directress
went to the Somme, and was installed with a staff of French
nurses in a huge field hospital of four thousand beds.

When the offensive in Champagne was started in April
1917, she undertook similar and, if possible, even more
arduous work in that region, winning for her intrepid
services the *Médaille des Épidémies*, the *Croix de Guerre*
(*avec palme*), and the Légion d'Honneur. Latterly the field
hospital in Belgium has been enlarged to eight hundred
beds. The latest Directress of this hospital has also won
the *Croix de Guerre*.

The Scottish Women's Hospital at Royaumont was
already a witness to the endurance of that ancient tie
between France and Scotland. And in this September a
new link was added in Paris itself, by the formation of the
Hôpital de l'Écosse in the Rue de la Chaise. This was already
before the war a well-known nursing home of high repute,
the clinique of a distinguished French doctor. But in this
September it took the name of the *Hôpital de l'Écosse*, as
it was now to be supported by funds from Scotland. After
being financed for a time from Canada, it was taken over
by the Scottish branch of the British Red Cross Society.

The same month of September saw the opening of a hospital not far from Paris, at Ris-Orangis, in the Seine et Oise
Department, founded in the previous July by two English
donors. The building offered to the founders by the French
Government was a disused college of the Marist Fathers.
As it had not been occupied for ten years, and had no
modern conveniences, a drastic overhauling of the whole
building was required. Every room was painted afresh, and

fitted with hot-water radiators. Electric light, gas, and water were laid on. Not only this, but baths, wash-basins, and sinks had all to be provided, and an entirely new system of sanitation installed. All this was done with magnificent thoroughness, and in a very short space of time the hospital was ready for the arrival of the first patients.

The hospital is fortunate in being surrounded by a park of forty acres. But ten years of disuse and neglect had produced a wild profusion of weeds and undergrowth, and paths which were choked with tangle, roads which had become obliterated, had to be found and cleared. When this work had been done, gravel paths and concrete terraces were revealed, most useful for the patient who is in need of sun and air. The Gate-House, which had fallen into ruin, was repaired and put in order; and it now houses the male staff of the hospital – sixty and more in number.

The *Hôpital Militaire* V.R. 76, as the unit at Ris-Orangis is formally called, is distinguished by the special excellence and completeness of its technical equipment. The X-Ray department, fitted out in the minutest detail, and the bacteriological laboratory have been able to further and facilitate the work of the surgeons to an exceptional degree, and to collect a mass of valuable data. The hospital has also been noted for the development, under a famous New York surgeon, who has given his voluntary services, of the system of suspensory treatment for fractures, widely adopted during the war. Instead of being put in plaster, the limb is suspended by an arrangement of pulleys and weights. This not only gives comfort to the patient, allowing him to move about in bed, and greatly reducing the pain, but enables the dressings to be done much more easily and with less risk of injury, since the limb is approachable from every direction. Moreover, the neighbouring joints are not immobilised, and as soon as the bone joins, the patient can often use his limb at once.

Recognising the high efficiency of the hospital, with its wonderful completeness of outfit, the French *Service de Santé* has made it the surgical and radiographical centre for a circuit of six military hospitals in the neighbourhood.

The motor section, which consists of a fleet of fourteen cars, collects and evacuates the wounded not only for this circuit of six hospitals, as well as for Ris-Orangis itself, but for six other hospitals in addition. The wounded arrive by train at Villeneuve St-Georges, a railway junction some miles away, where a canteen has been established, and the men supplied with hot or cooling drinks on arrival. Here the English staff allots the wounded men to the various hospitals in the district of which Ris-Orangis is the centre; the worst cases are reserved for Ris-Orangis itself.

A few days after this one-time college of the Marist Fathers began to receive its first wounded, a hospital was opened at the Château St-Rome, far away in the south-west of France, in the neighbourhood of Toulouse.

Château St-Rome is the home of the *Présidente* of the *Comité Britannique* and her husband. It stands in its park in the broad airy valley of the Garonne, within sight of the distant Pyrenees. At the opening of the war it was placed by its owners at the disposal of the Government for use as a hospital, but at that time the Government did not avail itself of the offer. In the summer of 1915, however, a request was made for the use of the château; and the hospital opened on 2nd October. It has three hundred beds, distributed among buildings surrounding the château.

Hôpital Complémentaire No. 54 (St-Rome's official title)

is peculiar in this, that it is the only *Hôpital Complément-aire* run, at the direct request of the *Service de Santé*, by an entirely British staff of doctors and nurses. The *Service de Santé* finances the unit, but it has had great help from England, especially from the *Comité Britannique*.

When it first opened, St-Rome received convoys of wounded from the front.; later on, they came from the interior. In December of 1916 it was chosen to be a special hospital for wounded suffering from chronic osteitis. Compound fractures failing to heal result in this condition, and such cases are particularly difficult and prolonged; but they have been treated at St-Rome with great success.

In November a hospital of five hundred beds was opened at St-Cloud in wooden buildings provided by the French. It is the Canadian General Hospital No. 8, and is staffed by the CAMC.

1916-1917

On New Year's Day 1916, the Edinburgh and Border and Border Hospital, originally at Malo-les-Bains, by Dunkirk, was reopened at Paris in the Bois de Boulogne. A restaurant in a leafy part of the Bois was transformed in a fortnight. Sanitary arrangements were put in at heavy cost. With its pleasant surroundings, the Pavilion Royal makes an admirable hospital for the seriously wounded cases, for which it is reserved. There are eight fully trained English nurses, and four V.A.Ds. The surgeons are French; and the hospital is under the direction of the *Service de Santé*.

In September of this year the Michelham Hospital, lodged in the Astoria Hotel, Paris, was reorganised, and since that date has had French patients and a mostly British staff. During the first year of the war this hospital took in British wounded, and had a mixed French and English staff. For the second year it had French patients and a Japanese staff. French ladies help. There are 183 beds in this hospital.

In July a hospital at Troyes was taken over from the French by the Canadian AMC, and became No. 6 General Canadian Hospital. It has 1400 beds for French wounded.

Two new hospitals opened during 1916 were both small hospitals for particular kinds of convalescent cases.

The first is the one already referred to, which was established at Martouret by the same lady who had started the hospital at Céret in the previous year. It is officially named Établissement de l'Assistance aux Convalescents Militaires Français (Fondation Allhusen No. 2).

Martouret is an old bathing establishment close to the little town of Die in the Dauphiné Alps. It stands by itself on a hill fifteen hundred feet up, in a beautiful country. The hospital was opened at the end of May; and because of the properties of the resinous baths it was asked to specialise in nerve cases and cases of rheumatism. Recently convalescent cases of malaria, so frequent among the soldiers from Salonika, have also been admitted. There are forty-five beds. The hospital is under the administration of the Lyons Région; and the wounded come from centres like Valence, Lyons, Grenoble, Aix-les-Bains, and Chambéry.

The second hospital was officially opened on 19th November, at Carqueiranne, in the Department of Var. This has special interest of having been built expressly as a sanatorium by the well-known Anglo-Swedish lady who founded and directs it. Her particular object was to do something for those soldiers whom long exposure, the wet cold of the trenches, and the hardships of winter campaigning, or the after-effects of chest and throat wounds, have predisposed to tuberculosis, or in whom some lung trouble has been set up which without special treatment will develop into that disease. There was, and is, a very real need for sanatoria of this kind, where timely and suitable treatment saves the sufferers' lives. The Sanatorium Beau-soleil is a white building, long and low, standing on a pine-grown hill beside the Mediterranean. It is sheltered from cold winds, takes all the sun, and has the scent of herbs and flowers about it. It has room for thirty patients. The land and means for building were provided out of a fund left to the foundress for this purpose by an Englishwoman who had married a French nobleman; but valuable help in carrying out and supporting the scheme was given by the *Comité Britannique* and by private subscribers in England. The patients are chosen by the Assistance aux Convalescents Militaires, a society attached to the French War Office, which has co-operated in the scheme from the first. The appreciation of the Government was shown by its sending a Minister to open the sanatorium at a function brilliant with notable persons.

In December the Argyll-Robertson Maison de Convalescence was opened in a villa at Dinan in Brittany, with thirty beds.

In January 1917 a French hospital at Port-à-Binson, in the Marne Department, *Hôpital Auxiliaire* No. 76, was taken over by the First Aid Nursing Yeomanry Corps. Some account of this Corps has been given in the story of the convoys. After the closing of the hospital maintained by the Corps at Calais for Belgian wounded in October 1916, an urgent request was made by the French for the FANY to take over the hospital at Port-à-Binson. The building, a priory, was inspected, and an agreement was made. The FANY was to supply nurses, chauffeurs, cars, and one hundred beds, with bedding, material and stores. Rations, light, and heating were to be provided by the *Société de Secours aux Blessés Militaires*. On 14th January 1917, a telegram arrived at Calais, asking for the cars and staff to start at once. In two or three hours three cars had begun their three-hundred-mile journey in the midst of a snow-storm; and others followed the next day. There were some breakdowns and consequent stoppages in lonely places in the snow. But in a few days all had arrived at Binson. Here there was much cleaning to be done; and the hospital was not formally opened till March, when the wards appeared not only clean, but dainty and attractive to the eye. The grounds are ample, and the place looks out on a fine prospect, with southern sun. Two French doctors divided the surgical work. Two refugee nuns looked after the linen room, and other nuns at a farmhouse did the washing. Apart from these and the orderlies the staff was all English. As the result of inspections and reports, the hospital was appointed to be a Triage (sorting) centre for the whole army in that district.

In January 1918, the FANY was asked to hand over the hospital to the *Société de Secours aux Blessés Militaires*.

Lastly we have to record the opening, in the first days of October 1917, of the *Hôpital Néo-Zélandais* at Étrembières, Haute Savoie.

This is a hospital for *rapatriés*; that is, refugees from the invaded and devastated regions of France, who, after being detained in Germany, are returned to their own country through Switzerland. We shall have more to say about the *rapatriés* when we come to speak of the relief work for refugees undertaken by the Society of Friends. That Society has a convalescent home at Samoëns in the same neighbourhood.

The hospital at Étrembieres was built in 1877 as a school for girls, and stands in a beautiful park at the foot of a mountain called the Salève. It is about three miles from Geneva, and just within French territory. The New Zealand Government has generously endowed the hospital, and it is managed by the British Committee of the French Red Cross.

The building was found to adapt itself fairly well to use as a hospital, providing eight large wards and two or three small ones, with accommodation for three hundred to three hundred and fifty patients. The staff, both doctors and nurses, is entirely British. Every variety of disease and injury can be treated here, as there is an operating theatre, sterilising room, dental and electrical departments, etc.

Two trains, one in the morning, and the other in the evening, arrive at Évian on the frontier bringing the *rapatriés* – eight hundred to a thousand of them at a time. They have lost home, possessions, everything. Now they are on the soil of France, they have the friendliness of their own tongue in their ears; but they are still homeless and still among strangers in a land that to them is strange. They are still exiles from their own villages and familiar countryside, which they see in memory scorched with fires and pounded with shells; which they know are still in the hands of a merciless invader; and which, when at last they are permitted to go home, they will find defaced and pillaged or mere ash and blackened ruin. No wonder that when they emerge from the train at Évian they look round them on the Savoy mountains with dazed eyes.

The healthy among them are sent on by train and distributed over France. The sick are examined on their arrival by doctors, who detain them for a night or two, and then draft them into various hospitals in the neighbourhood, of which the Néo-Zélandais is the largest.

The *rapatriés* are absolutely homeless. Families therefore cannot be separated. If one of a family is sick and goes to hospital, the rest must go as well. For adults a lodging is found in the neighbouring village. The children are put in a villa which stands in the grounds of the hospital. There they are taught and trained in household management, by a little band of nuns.

This concludes the list of the Anglo-French hospitals, that is, hospitals for French wounded staffed and controlled from Britain or the British Dominions. As the reader may remember, however, much work has been done in purely French hospitals by groups and individuals. Nearly all this work has been nursing; but surgeons also have gone out from this country and given their services. For example, at the hospital of Lamothe (*Hôpital* 115 bis, Villeneuve-sur-Lot) in the Department of Lot et Garonne, British surgeons have been working. In the autumn of 1914 an urgent appeal was made by the British Committee of the French Red Cross for British surgeons to help in the work of this hospital centre. Ever since, a service has been assured by one or more surgeons, who work not only in the hospital, but in the surrounding district, and have indeed acted as consulting surgeons to the seventeen other hospitals of this 'région.' This voluntary service has been warmly appreciated by the French.

Of the labours of the nurses, it is, of course, impossible to give any detailed account, dispersed as they have been in so many quarters. But a brief description of the fortunes of one of these small English units may be given, as fairly typical experience.

The unit in question attached itself to a military hospital at Foix, officially named *Hôpital Temporaire* No. 1 (Ariège). It was a large hospital of over five hundred beds. The expedition was something of a venture.

'It was in December 1914,' writes one of these ladies, the unit's leader, 'that we started for Foix, knowing nothing but that a French doctor had said that he would be glad to have us, and that Foix was the kind of place no one else would want to go to.

'Our arrival must still be remembered – narrow climbing streets, dark half Spanish houses, crowding peasants who whispered in amazement, "*Les Inglès!*" and then the huge gloomy hospital, packed with wounded, comfortless, dingy, dreary beyond all words. Green and chocolate paint, still wet after twenty years, floors dark with dirt, walls streaked with damp, dust in all the corners, and in the untidy, sunless wards those rows of silent men staring dully at the ceiling. One felt one would do anything in the world to change the look on their faces. But there were only five of us; we had no equipment (all the cleaning materials for my eighty-five beds were one chipped enamel basin and the bottom of a pair of soldier's trousers), and the one friendly doctor was called away a few days after our arrival. The rest of the staff eyed us with suspicion; all that we did was "*trés étrange*" and when we wanted to give a rubber hot water bottle to a patient instead of a stone one, the *infirmier de visite* had first to consult the doctor... The tables and trays had to be scraped with a knife and the men spoke of the last time they had been washed as one speaks of "last Christmas" or "a little before Easter." It was not any one's fault exactly; the country was very poor and very remote, the *Service de Santé* had been overwhelmed by the great September rush, and staff was lacking or inexperienced; but courage often failed us, there seemed such walls of suspicion and misunderstanding to break down. Only the men cheered us on. They gave us immediately blind confidence and unfailing respect. The hopeless look went out of their faces, and they cared to live because we cared so dreadfully that they should not die. They were very amused at us of course, and spent their time guessing what form of energy we would next display; but when even the orderlies became enthusiastic and the *Médecin-chef* found that our wards were the best disciplined and the men the happiest, he accepted us as part of the hospital, and whenever Inspectors or Generals came, we were hurriedly rounded up and proudly presented to them as "*son équipe anglaise.*"

'It was a great satisfaction when he asked whether more helpers would not be able to come, and soon our number had increased to fourteen, all voluntary, with nothing but war experience, but very keen, very adaptable, very happy to work for France. After a time other hospitals in the XVII. Région hinted that they too would like "*les dames anglaises,*" and the *Directeur du Service de Santé* asked me to visit any of their hospitals which I thought might be in need of nurses, as parts of the region were very poor, and there was little local help to be obtained.

'Soon Pamier's three hospitals (420 beds in all) had a small band of nurses, and in Saint-Gaudens (300 beds) one solitary Englishwoman worked miracles of energy and skill. In 1915, Saint-Rome (300 beds) was entirely staffed by English doctors and nurses, and the French authorities themselves flew a Union Jack over their own military building side by side with the French flag.

'Later on Salies-du-Salat (100 beds for surgical tuberculosis) asked also for an English staff, which has been a great success.

'Through the unfailing generosity of British and American Committees, chiefly perhaps through the *Comité Britannique*, we were able to do much for the comfort of the men and to help in the saving of their lives. What had begun as a most humble and private venture developed into quite an important undertaking, and it says much for the tact and discretion of the English nurses that the *Service de Santé* should have welcomed them so eagerly into their own hospitals. In this lies the interest of the work, for I think we were the first to work only for the *Service de Santé* and not for the *Croix Rouge*. It was rather a difficult position sometimes, because there was never any "precedent" for the things we did; we must have broken all their rules a hundred times over, and we could never remember that administrations must not be hurried! But all the same, much courteous patience on their part and great goodwill on ours resulted in the most pleasant relations, and an appreciation which I hope was mutual. I know that on our side we could never be sufficiently grateful for the kindness shown to us, and for the honour of being allowed to serve the Army of France.'

The hospital at Salies-du-Salat, mentioned in this account, is in the Haute Garonne. When the English nurses first went there in November 1916, there were no nurses, and only Annamese orderlies speaking no French. A few months after the arrival of our nurses, the *Médecin-chef* put up a notice announcing that, owing to the improved discipline, longer leave and other privileges would be given. The small staff has done splendid work in face of much to dishearten, for the hospital is exclusively for cases of surgical tuberculosis, and the patients are all fairly far gone in the disease.

Another hospital for surgical tuberculosis is at Palavas, on the Mediterranean shores, near Montpellier; and here, too, is a staff of English V.A.D. nurses and a matron. The original party went out in the early summer of 1916. The Délégué of the British Committee of the French Red Cross in that région of France saw how great was the need of the hospital, which eagerly accepted the services of the English nurses.

Lastly, it must be mentioned that Australia, which has shown so spontaneous and generous a sympathy for France, has provided, through the Australian Branch of the British Red Cross Society, a unit of twenty fully trained nurses – and none are more skilled or highly trained – for work in the French hospitals. Through the *Comité Britannique* these nurses have been allocated in small units to hospitals all over France. These nurses of British race scattered among the French hospitals had a double mission. It has been theirs not only to nurse the sick and wounded soldiers; but they have also helped the new-born effort of France to raise the standard of the nursing profession, and win for it the public esteem which it enjoys in England.

As a pendant to the work of the hospitals, we may end with a word on the vans equipped for special work – radiography, dentistry, bacteriology – which have been sent out by the *Comité Britannique*.

Thirteen specially-constructed automobiles, equipped for X-Ray work, have been sent out. In the field hospitals close to the front it is impossible to have a fixed apparatus; but if the X-Rays can be used on the spot, it will often save both precious time and still more precious lives. Therefore this mobile service, arranged for by the *Comité Britannique* and the Headquarters Staff, has been of a value hard to overestimate. This work at the front is done by military operators.

The Dental Ambulances have also signally proved their worth. Two of these were sent out in the summer of 1916. They are solidly built vans of imposing size, seven feet broad, and weighing some four and a half tons. The design and fittings were the fruit of much careful thought, but only actual experience of French roads could test them thoroughly for the purpose in view, and in practice it was found that a few details had to be modified. On their side, the French – then in process of completing similar cars – adopted certain devices from these English ambulances, such as luggage nets, sleeping hammocks, water-tank and tent; while some ingenious French contrivances gave useful hints to the English. It was a case of mutual help. The

French *Service de Santé* had had an experimental dental van at the front for some months, and were then about to send out a fleet of them.

Trouble with teeth – often acute – is, of course, very common in every large army. The medical officers have not the necessary instruments for treating the sufferers, who cannot, on the other hand, be spared the time to go back to the base hospital. The trouble continues; the men cannot chew their food, and in consequence fall sick. There are also men whose artificial teeth get broken, and who are then helpless. This means a vast amount of pain and waste, which need not be with an adequate service of dental ambulances. The French have recognised that a mobile service is really a necessity, and have equipped and sent out a number of dental cars. As we have said, these were being completed, after successful experiment, with a car at the front, when the two English cars sent out through the *Comité Britannique* arrived in Paris. Each of the English cars has for crew or staff two dental surgeons and a mechanic. They left England at the beginning of July 1916 (just in time to meet the first batch of German prisoners from the Somme embarking on the other side), and after a rather protracted delay in Paris, received orders to start for an unknown destination. This proved to be somewhere on the Flanders front. They were attached to an Army Corps, and Dunkirk was appointed their headquarters. Operations were at last begun at a little ancient town some distance away from Dunkirk. Fifty patients were treated the first day. Extractions were performed in the tent, called by the soldiers '*la salle des bourreaux*,' and fillings in the car itself. It was the beginning of a campaign for which thousands of aching soldiers have been grateful.

The difficulty of having the necessary apparatus in field hospitals close to the front, presents itself again with regard to bacteriological work. A laboratory for this work is indispensable to a completely equipped base hospital to-day; but the lack of this precious adjunct in the front line and clearing hospitals often leads to a faulty diagnosis. A mobile laboratory is the only solution; and this the British Committee have had made and equipped in London, and sent to France on a motor-lorry chassis, in the summer of 1917. It was designed by a French Army bacteriologist, collaborating with one of the committee's own workers in France. A generous subscriber supplied the internal equipment, by which cases can be diagnosed and lives saved by instant inoculation or despatch to a special hospital. Arrived on the scene, the van expands, by sections neatly stowed, into a good-sized room, with windows, electric light, incubators, stoves, and all the hundred appliances for carrying out every kind of test. The French Medical Service had no funds voted for such experimental work, though an Army surgeon had the idea and the genius for working it out. Once again, the Red Cross could step in and prove its value.

We have pictured a day's routine in the office of the *Comité Britannique* in London. Let us now give a glimpse of the work-a-day life in an Anglo-French Hospital in France.

THE DAY OF AN ORDERLY

A hospital orderly fills a humble office. He is the unskilled labourer of the little world he moves in. He is at everybody's beck and call. There are no pedantic limitations to his duties: their variety is infinite. All odd jobs are his. If he starts to perform some part of his daily routine, it is ten to one that a Sister will waylay him with a request that cannot be put aside, and that diverging on his errand he will meet the Matron on the stairs with some yet more urgent commission, and that before he is half-way through with this the imperious call of the *Médecin-chef* will summon him to 'chuck that,' and demand his instant services elsewhere. He does not complain; on the contrary, he is inclined to become rather vain of being after all so indispensable a person.

Modest though his functions are, he has opportunities for observation. And perhaps on that account it may be worthwhile to try to picture for the reader a typical day in the life of an orderly. If the following lines are written in the first person, let it be understood that it is any orderly who speaks.

But first it must be explained that the particular hospital in which our orderly describes his day has its own special organisation. In many of the hospitals with which this book is concerned – I think in most of them – the duties of the orderly are performed by French soldiers. But at the Chateau of A—— the orderlies are all English volunteers. At home in England they are engaged in various blameless and elegant occupations – build houses and churches, paint pictures, write books, adorn perhaps the Civil Service; but here they come to bed-rock matters and explore fundamental things. Our orderly, however, shall speak for himself. The year is 1916, the month is June.

It is close on nine o'clock in the morning, and I am sweeping the steps of the château that lead down into the park. The sun is already hot, and reflects a glare from the white stone.

There is no particular necessity to sweep the steps, but it is odd what pleasure one can take in this simple ritual, and it fills a few moments between breakfast and the real labours of the day. On each side of the wide stairs is a rose tree, one red and one yellow. Other sweepers of steps may belong to a different school; but I always allow a few of the scattered petals – they are single roses – to remain on the swept surface.

Beyond a broad stretch of gravel – there is nothing in the way of a garden to intervene – the grass begins, and as far as the eye can see the level park spreads its verdure, narrowing in the hazy distance where a ridge of hill curves to enclose it in steep woods. Single trees, and clumps, are dotted over the green; and here and there little wooden bridges mark the course of shallow trout-streams.

Quite close, and nearly opposite the steps, is a great tulip tree; and round its stem a shelter has been constructed – an umbrella-shaped roof, under which are a quantity of *chaises longues* for the wounded. Two are lounging there already, in pyjamas. One has a book, the other is coiled up asleep.

At my left again, there is another shelter, a penthouse of wood built against the wall of the château. Pine boughs have been laid on the felt-covered roof of it, to mitigate the heat of the sun. Here are half a dozen beds, a little outdoor ward for patients whom the fresh air will help to recovery. From the steps, as I sweep, I can look down into the shelter, and I bid good-morning to my friends there, and ask what night they have had. It is not my turn, but one of my comrade's, to attend on the wounded of the *Abri*. Otherwise it would have been mine to bring them their coffee at seven and help the Sister with the breakfast and other after-breakfast duties. And I am glad, because I am still rather sleepy. It was four in the morning before I got to bed.

Yesterday afternoon the telephone bell rang. We were expecting a convoy, and it was no surprise to hear the voice from the station at B—— announcing that the train would arrive at our station, farther down the line, at eleven-thirty. Being familiar with these announcements, we are doubtful about that eleven-thirty. But the train must be met at that hour, though we may have to wait till morning at the station. I am one of those told off to go with the ambulances. Eighteen *blessés* are expected: four ambulances, and a touring car. We hope that two will be able to sit up in the car, otherwise – or if more than eighteen arrive – it will mean a second journey.

Sixteen stretchers must be got ready, and four blankets for each man. The French stretchers – lighter than English ones – have the canvas at one end raised to support the head, so a pillow is not required.

At eleven the cars are purring in the courtyard. Silence and sleep have descended on the hospital, where only the night nurses move in the shaded light. The stretchers are thrust in, and we start in procession. I sit beside the driver, who in normal life lectures at Cairo to the studious youth of Egypt, but here alternates the functions of chauffeur and assistant radiographer. We glide through the silent village and climb a long ascent. The head-lamps illuminate the ghostly green of endless ash-trees bordering the road; then the shuttered houses of a sleeping hamlet. The air strikes cold as we race along the upland. At last in the distance one sees the signal lights of the station. There is a level-crossing to be passed, and a drowsy porter slowly opens the gates as the waiting cars throb in line. A curve brings us to the station. The ambulances are backed on to it, the hoods thrown open, the stretchers and blankets got out.

We bring the stretchers into the station and pile them on the platform, for they will be taken on by the train in exchange for those on which the wounded arrive. There is an hour or more to wait. The hot milk and the water-bottles are kept warm at the stove in the little waiting-room. Some of us stretch ourselves on the platform benches, others sit on the platform edge and smoke. At last the train approaches in the darkness, glides almost imperceptibly into the station, and stops. *Infirmiers* hoist out the wounded allotted to us. As they deposit them on the platform on their stretchers, we carry them off to the waiting-room as fast as we can. In a few minutes each has had his hot drink or lemonade, has been inspected by the doctor, and has been lifted into the ambulance. The drinks are administered by the wife of our radiographer, who, like her husband, is an accomplished artist, but for the time being looks after the clothes and linen.

Two large lanterns set on the ground outside the main door of the château make a fantastic light in the courtyard as the cars, one after one, draw up silently opposite the door. The lantern-rays illuminate the lower branches of the limetrees by the courtyard wall, and cast a monstrous shadow from the cars on the dim foliage above. The hoods are thrown back, and we draw out, carefully and gently, the wounded on their stretchers, and lay them down in the porch. The doctor allots each to his ward, and we carry them up as rapidly as possible. In each hushed ward the Sister stands ready to receive them. A few heads are turned in curiosity to see the new inmates. But most are sound asleep. It is a relief to feel that at last their journey is over, and the agonising jolts of the road are behind them.

The vivid night scene is recollected like a dream, now that the June sun is radiant over the peaceful park. The cool shade of leafy trees over the stream is welcome as I dip my straw besom in the golden-tinted water. Returning, I hear a voice calling a name in friendly but peremptory tones. It is a nurse at a window in one of the lower wards summoning a patient from the park for the dressing of his wound. He comes, unwillingly, cherishing his bandaged arm.

And now our real work begins. Nine o'clock is the hour for the first operation. Two of my comrades have already brought the patient down the stairs, and are pushing him supine on a trolley along the passage to the theatre. There they will don a white robe and assist the surgeons and Sister.

Opposite the theatre is the X-Ray room, and each of the new arrivals has to pass the X-Rays this morning. We get our list of the men, in the order in which they are to be taken; take stretchers, and set to work. While one man is in the dark-room, which hums and splutters with sparks, as the radiographers prepare their magical apparatus, another waits on his stretcher in the passage – for there is no time to lose if we are to finish by noon – and we, the two bearers, give him a cigarette and talk.

Forty-eight hours ago, perhaps, or less, this man was lying out on the churned and shattered slopes of the Mort Homme or Côte 304. Some will have lain many hours, even a whole day or more, before they could be picked up. I marvel at their fortitude and elasticity. After a brief sleep and a meal they are amazingly revived, though nearly all are seriously wounded.

The men we are getting now are mostly Territorials, between thirty and forty in age, who have been flung into the furnace of Verdun. And splendidly have they quitted themselves. These solid, sunburnt, quiet men – no light weight on a stretcher – seem to belong to the very core of the nation which so indomitably and tenaciously is holding the gate of France against the colossal blows of the German armies. They are taciturn, with gentle voices; but they will stand to the last for 'all they have and are,' they will flinch from no suffering or calamity to save their beloved country. It is for them mere matter of course. Yet they hate the war.

Some show a mild curiosity and interest at finding themselves in an English hospital; most take it all for granted. One tells me he comes from the Doubs, another from the Indre; another, tall and heavy, is a farmer from Normandy; another is from the far south and grows fruit; he tells me he would like to get in touch with the English market, and wonders if I could help him. And so on. Different types, with widely different speech. The patois requires some patience to understand sometimes, and the French is often cheeringly ungrammatical to a foreign ear. The majority are *cultivateurs*, with a passion for their native soil inbred in blood and bone.

As each man comes out from the X-Ray examination, he is shifted from the table to the stretcher, and two bearers carry him back to his bed, while the other two bearers take up the man who is waiting, and he in his turn is shifted from the stretcher to the table on which he lies to be examined. We go to and from the wards, where the nurses are busy with the daily dressings of the wounds. Sometimes we meet a little procession returning from an operation with the patient still insensible or just emerging into consciousness, or else carrying off the next to be operated on, clutching the *fiche* which records his name and wound, amid the parting jokes and encouragements of his comrades.

The operating-table is universally known as *le billard*. The other day this little colloquy was heard, as a man was going to his seventh operation. '*Quoi? encore pour le billard?*' '*Mais, tu sais que je suis un abonne!*' And the victim went off with a smile and a waving hand. But now and then there is one who has a horror of the chloroform, as if there were some sinister magic in it.

Almost all, as soon as they are under the anæsthetic, go back to the battlefield; and you will hear sometimes the yell of the charge: '*Courage, les gars! En avant, la baionette!*' and the soldiers, hearing the cry ring out through the window, will listen with a kind of fascination. 'That's just how it is when we attack,' they will say.

The morning passes quickly. While we wait by our stretchers in the passage, we have an appearance of idleness, which is irresistible to Sisters who look out from their wards for someone to do one of the score of little errands in their repertory. Sometimes, when the X-rays promise a prolonged search for 'foreign bodies,' I yield to the blandishing request:

'Would you mind going down to the carpenters' shop?

I want...' or, 'Would you go and fetch the *Médecin-chef?*'
or, 'Could you get someone to mend my Primus stove?
It is always going out.' But if I do yield, and run down
to the carpenters, for instance, the shout of 'Orderly' will
inevitably echo down the corridor, and I fly back to my
post, leaving an unwelcomed and not too coherent message
behind me.

The carpenters are orderlies too. They work underground
in a stone cellar lighted by gratings which look out on
the courtyard. And very necessary functionaries they are
in the hospital's economy. For the château, stripped of its
own furniture, is a bare interior, and there are a hundred
things which have to be made on the spot – tables, cupboards, shelves, special splints, fracture-beds, etc. Fortu-
nately we are abundantly supplied with wood from the
saw-mill up the river. There have been dynasties in the
carpenters' shop. Little tables and other creations – works
of faith and enthusiasm – of the first and second dynasties are still extant, though bow-legged and apt to resolve
into their elements if not tenderly handled. But now we
have become imposingly proficient. A year ago I, myself,
the completest of amateurs, would spend my spare time
constructing little tables for the bedside of the wounded.
They were my pride and delight. They stood square. They
held things. But now, I can but gaze with awe on the
beautifully jointed constructions which our head carpenter
(he illustrates books in private life) makes with such care
and cunning – singular erections, destined to suspend by
cords and pulleys the broken limbs of patients, the latest
method of treating fractures.

Twelve o'clock. It is the hour for dinner. We have hurried
our last case to bed, and assemble in the great stone kitchen

in the basement, where the chef, a French soldier, presides over the steaming dishes.

For each *salle* there is a dish of meat and another of vegetables; and these we carry upstairs to their destination, where the portions are served out by the Sisters. The meat is usually a stew of beef. Occasionally it is wild boar, when one of them has been shot in the forest; or venison, when a *chevreuil* has been killed. (One night one of our cars coming down the hill ran full tilt into a deer that had chosen to go to sleep in the middle of the lonely road.) But it is not every patient who has a stomach for strong meats. Some have appetites that must be coaxed; and for these there are eggs, chicken, rabbit, sweetbreads, or fresh trout from the river. These special dishes we come back for, and hurry with them to the waiting Sisters. There is much coming and going up and down the dark stairway to the kitchen. The wine has already been distributed. This is a task that falls for a period to each orderly in turn.

He reigns in the cellar, a dark and humid place, where by the light of a tallow candle stump he fills each morning the prescribed number of bottles, apportioning exactly a certain quantity to each of the wards, different in each case, as the number of beds varies. When a cask is finished, he heaves a new one to its settle and broaches it; and when the hospital is full, this happens pretty often. The wine when given out is mixed with water, to the disgust of the soldiers, who are all firmly persuaded that *le vin donne de la force*, and that water is a dangerous drink.

It generally happens that there are some patients who cannot feed themselves. There is one lying in the window, a bearded man who is flat on his back with his right arm stretched out at right angles in a splint. And in another ward is a boy who has lost an eye since he came in, and both whose hands are full of wounds and tied up. He put up his hands to save his face when the shell burst. (He is one of a family of thirteen, very poor, and worked on a canal boat in the region of Dunkirk.) If there is time, we take a turn with the nurses, who have all they can do to serve the full wards, in feeding poor fellows like these. They contrive to make some amusement out of their helplessness. But in a few minutes it is time to fetch the sweets. And when these are despatched, there are the empty dishes, plates, etc., to be carried down in big baskets.

Those of the wounded who can move about help in distributing the food, and wash up the glasses after the meal. There is a brown Arab boy, in a fez and loose scarlet jacket, who moves about in a silent, smiling way; he is very deft with his one free hand.

Now it is time to dispose of the pails of slops and dressings, which means several journeys up and down stairs. And then, with the few inevitable odd jobs that arise, the morning's work is done. But going down to wash for dinner I notice that something has happened in the hall below the front staircase. It is no longer empty, but crowded with huge bales and packages. More work for orderlies! But appetite calls first. Dinner is somewhat indefinite in its beginning and end, as there is always work to keep some of us late or to call them away early. The *Directrice* of the hospital sits at one end of the long table, the *Médecin-chef* at the other. Post has arrived in the morning, and the last news from England is discussed, along with the trivial affairs that amuse our small community. Sugar has become excessively scarce – otherwise food is plentiful enough – and the sweet-toothed among us are driven to secrete little *caches* of precious lumps in odd nooks and corners, which of course are considered legitimate booty by raiding rivals; scenes of triumph and consternation ensue. But sometimes we are on our best behaviour, when generals or high officers on a tour of inspection, with crimson velvet breeches and khaki tunics, deign to be our guests, and compliments ripple across the table.

The meal over, the question of 'carrying out' arises. If it is fine, we carry out into the garden as many of the wounded as want, or are allowed, to go. A few have been already carried out this morning, in the intervals of other work. The weather is not too settled; will it rain this afternoon? Having decided that it will not, we sort ourselves in pairs; each pair takes a stretcher, and we attack the different *salles* in turn.

It is surprising what a difference sun and air and the change from the sameness of the ward to a large and living horizon works on the men, though some, in their languor and exhaustion, are at first unwilling to be moved. Here, in one of the upper wards, is a youth with pallid face, whom the nurses can hardly persuade to touch his food, and who shrinks from the slightest movement. With his dreamy eyes and dark close-curling hair and little beard, he has the least military appearance in the world. Yet I find he has not only the *Croix de Guerre* but the *Médaille Militaire* – corresponding to our Victoria Cross – and has done deeds of signal gallantry. But I am no longer surprised, for such cases are frequent, and one gets more and more experience of the splendid unexpectedness of human nature. This romantic-looking youth, who in a week will have regained his colour and his appetite out of doors, tells me how he and his comrades were sent to learn bomb-throwing with the British Third Army. In this art our proficiency in games enables us for once to be teachers. But that, after all, is but a small return for what the French have taught us in artillery.

If just a few are reluctant to go, most of the men are impatient to be out, and lively reproaches assail us from this bed or that when anything has delayed our coming. They become expert in throwing themselves from bed to stretcher, having found ways of their own of transferring their wounded limbs without injury. But certain cases have to be moved ever so gingerly, with the most elaborate precautions and many groans. There are four or five who cannot be moved to a stretcher, and these have to be carried down on their beds. There are no lifts in the chateau, needless to say; and to carry a loaded bed downstairs, keeping it level all the time, is not the lightest of jobs, but with four bearers it is accomplished quite quickly.

For those who have been perhaps six or seven months in the ward the ' first day out ' is a long-looked-for occasion, a memorable date. One seems to feel with them the wonder of delicious sunshine and rustling leaves, and the life-giving sweetness of the air.

With all the speed we can, we come and go, till we have some thirty laid at ease on *chaises longues* under the tulip-tree, or in a smaller group under an apple-tree near the stream. As many more perhaps can walk, and are now lying on the grass, or under more distant trees, or strolling by the little river. Now and then a group will play at bowls on the gravel. It will be the fashion for a week or two, but enthusiasm for games is apt to flicker out. One day we got up a match between the different wards; only *couchés* – those who could not walk – being admitted to compete. The occasion of the match was this. There was a certain patient, whom we will call No. 43, who lay in his bed for months and made no progress, in great measure because he refused all effort towards recovery and englobed himself in a mental and corporeal apathy. He was a young man, but without an attribute of youth. He was a soldier, but no one ever looked less like one. Pallid, with fixed, expressionless brown eyes, he remained in a sort of jellied vacancy. Sometimes his parents would visit him; and it was a sight at once pitiable and absurd to see this short, stout, sable-attired pair hovering with fish-like, tearful eyes over their cherished offspring. No. 43 was the despair of the doctors. These were on the point of trying if an application of electricity might succeed in shaking him from the glue of passivity in which he seemed fixed and imbedded for ever, when someone hit on the notion of the match of bowls. The champions were carried out on their stretchers, and from their supine position flung the bowls forward. And No. 43, invigorated by a sort of resentment at being roused into activity, won the match. We crowned him with laurels. He was seen to smile. One of our comrades, noted for his joyous and irreverent badinage, rallied him on the festive revelries and boisterous escapades which he felt sure had marked his roseate youth. No. 43 resumed his ox-like solemnity of visage, and replied in a sentence of finished prose: '*Monsieur, j'ai assisté à des réunions de toutes sortes; et je me suis toujours contenu entre les limites les plus correctes.*'

But 43 was altogether an exception among the wounded. Who so ready with a merry word about their sufferings, who so prompt with a cordial and engaging smile, who so grateful for the least attention, as these soldiers of France? And what elasticity they have, both of mind and body! They do not want to be helped too much when first regaining the use of their limbs; they are eager to help themselves. They are often even too eager at the first trial of their crutches, and hop about with reckless agility. Then comes a day when the crutches are discarded. They are still very weak; but one of us walks behind with a firm grip of the jacket or pyjamas between the shoulders in case of a tumble; and they descend the stairs with increasing confidence, turning round with a triumphant smile to say: *'J'ai fait du progrès, n'est-ce-pas?'*

There are three men whom we have carried out who are liable to haemorrhage at any instant. The outing is excellent for them, but they cause us anxious moments. We have laid them nearer to the château than the rest, and a watchful eye is kept on them, for if the alarm is called they must be carried to the operating theatre with lightning speed. At present, however, they seem to be perfectly at ease, and we hope for the best.

Now is the time for a pleasant lounge and chat with the wounded, some of whom are now old friends. But there are those packing-cases in the hall, crying out to be opened. A swift ripping up of the canvas discloses the contents of the bales. There are bandages, gauze, lint – all sorts of hospital stores – shirts, socks, slippers, etc., sent out by the *Comité Britannique* from Knightsbridge. Long awaited private parcels too, for the staff, are eagerly pounced on and carried off; and other big packages from the country town where our shopping and provisioning are done. We have a busy time carrying one load to the top of the house, superintended by the Matron, another to the pharmacy, another to the *épicerie*. I realise, as never before, the weight of jam.

The, last load is disposed of, and a broom restores what our genial Vaguemestre and secretary, whose phrasing is as elegant as his handwriting, calls *le péristyle*, to a presentable cleanness of aspect.

It is from here that, when there has been a death, the little funeral procession starts to the church close by. I forbear to describe the grief of widow or parents summoned perhaps from some distant department of France. Many, both men and women, assemble to honour him who has died, and follow him to his grave in the cemetery on the outskirts of the village. It is the duty of two of us to follow, too, and under the tall trees on the hillside where the soldier is laid to rest, to represent the homage of England to the fallen son of France.

Three o'clock! I remember that ten men are being evacuated to-day, and that it falls to me to fit them out with such clothes and shoes as they may be in need of. Having a list of these men in my pocket, I proceed to collect them. When all have been assembled, I take them down in turn to a part of the spacious cellars where the clothing is stored. Each of the soldiers has already received the things taken from him when he came in, since disinfected and repaired; but one wants new trousers, another a jacket, a third a cap, and nearly all want boots. I fit them as best I can. Some take the first thing that comes, easily content. Others insist on trying one thing after another, and would reject them all if a further choice were possible. But what we have must serve. As it happens, all the smaller sized boots have been taken already; the new stock has not arrived; none but gigantic sizes are left; and all the men's feet are unnaturally small. I assure them that with some paper stuffed in the toes they will be admirably fitted. They shuffle about, make comical or dubious grimaces, but finally depart in a general good humour, all more or less pleased with the haphazard smartness of their variegated new get-up.

A few minutes' stroll among the wounded in the park, and we may snatch an interval for tea in company with Sisters and nurses. During the warm weather we have tea under a great horse-chestnut in a garden between the church tower and the river; a sunny, secluded spot.

Returning to the château, I meet someone on a bicycle, who hails me as he alights at the entrance. It is Gaston – one of last year's *blessés*, returned to pay us a visit. After many months in the hospital – how well I remember his weight on a stretcher – he had to lose his foot. But here he is, strong, tall, and upright, riding a bicycle! He has an artificial foot (American) and his limp is barely noticeable. It is delightful to see him again; and he is soon surrounded by old friends of the staff, as his arrival is noised about, eager with questions and hand-grasps.

But I am hastily summoned by a nurse on an errand from one of the upper wards. A young Arab, she tells me, who has just had his arm put in plaster, is trying to tear off his bandage and needs controlling. I find him, scarcely emerged from the effects of the anaesthetic, making resentful movements like a puzzled animal and every other moment laying out his throat for a blank roar. His mouth opens wide for a perceptible interval before the roar comes, and his eyes are frightened and angry. But one of my comrades is already in charge of him, and I am not really wanted. To-morrow the boy will be smiling and human again.

In the same ward are two *amputés* – middle-aged men – whom I can never pass without a twist of the heart. One has lost an arm, the other a leg. Their sad patience never gives way. Yesterday I stole a rose for each of them, and

I see the red bloom and the white still beside their beds, stuck in water. Their smile of thanks haunts me and hurts.

It will soon be time for carrying-in, and I go down to the wounded under the tulip-tree and sit among them. We exchange cigarettes and chat. They have all been greatly moved and impressed by the death of Kitchener. Vaguely they have felt the strength and stature of the man who raised our armies from the soil; and his passing from the world into the silence of those stormy waters at sunset in the far North has a legendary and mysterious grandeur for them. Moreover, he was a friend of France. But we talk of many things. They tell stories of the trenches at Verdun, blasted away by the infernal cannonade; of the smell of ether as the drugged Boches advanced and fell and came on again; fumes that hung over the heaps of dead. And we talk of our homes. But some have homes no longer. Here is a man from a village beyond Lille. He has a wife and children there, but knows nothing of what has become of them, only that they are in the power of the Boche. And here in the hospital he has had to lose a leg. But he speaks with a surprising gentleness. War is all very well, he tells me, for soldiers who can fight; but this making war on women and children, *vraiment, ce n'est pas bien*. Next him is a lad of twenty, who has been *téléphoniste* at a grand hotel in Paris. He has bad wounds; it will be a year or more, I think, before he has ended with hospitals, and his fighting days are over. He has the most winning of smiles, and he talks to me of London, where he has spent a week or two, and which he has a great desire to revisit. And truly I hope to see him there. Another who knows England, and indeed speaks admirable English, is coming towards us over the grass. He has several wounds, but comparatively slight ones, and is handsome, with aquiline dark features. He comes from Evreux in Normandy, and the wool trade takes him to England for long visits. He is happy to have come to an English hospital. But, for the most part, these soldiers are as ignorant of our country as the men of our army, before the war's experience, were of France. They find that Englishwomen are merrier than Frenchwomen; but I don't know that this surprised them.

I doubt if they had any prejudices on the subject. The other day I found a whole group who believed that India was a part, or a continuation, of Turkey. And perhaps if one could see into their minds, their ideas of England and the English would be found to be equally fabulous. But they ask many questions, always a little puzzled at first that we should come here of our own accord to work for France, when there was no compulsion to do so. They are quick to note character, and the human comedy in our little community does not escape them. On the other side of the tree is a sallow Corsican, who worked in the engine-room of a tramp steamer. We talk of the wonders of New York, where he means to live when the war is over. But he is a complainer, this Corsican, though he can talk pleasantly enough – he likes to use his Italian – and he is not a favourite in the ward. Next him is a soft-voiced, bright-eyed youth, who works in a grocery in Limoges; and there is a vinegrower from the Rhone Valley, and a long-faced silent Norman; and not far off is a man with clear brown eyes and a short moustache who, to my surprise, turned out to be a cure from Dijon. In a little separate group is D——, a sergeant and old soldier, who has about him the air of tradition, as if he were truly a descendant of the *Grande Armée* of a hundred years ago. I greatly enjoy his company; he is a man of no flow of speech, though he comes from the Midi; but he is so genuine a man, so fine of feeling, reserved as he is, so loyal, to use a word the French are fond of, so frank and cordial in his simplicity, that one feels it good to be with him. I found him once discussing art and letters – an unusual thing among the *blessés* – with a little black-haired, heavy-moustached soldier, who, in other times, is a dealer in curios and pictures in Paris. He, too, is a man of excellent heart and intelligence, though I was a little disconcerted when our talk happened on the theatre and Shakespeare. D—— had not heard of Shakespeare, and my other friend, a little scandalised, proceeded to explain that he was the '*Victor Hugo de l'Angleterre*' – and the famous author of *Quo Vadis*?

Germans of a similar walk in life would, I doubt not, possess more instruction. But how often will you find a German middle-class family priding themselves on having read Goethe and Shakespeare and Kant, but apparently quite unaffected by the culture they have passed through their minds and still essentially boorish, still capable of a yet greater pride in the capacity for drinking twelve glasses of beer between meals! These Frenchmen, even the illiterate peasant, have always natural dignity and grace of speech.

And now I hear my name called by a Breton lad, bright-eyed and round-headed, with short black hair and a little black moustache, white teeth, and a roguish laugh. He has just waked up from a nap, and insists that I shall take a walk with him in the park after supper. Already the stretchers are being brought out, and I join with the others in carrying the soldiers indoors. We get this done at a great speed, and soon there are only a few loiterers left who need no help. The hæmorrhages have refrained from hæmorrhaging, and all is well.

At six o'clock we muster again in the kitchen to carry up the supper for the wounded – usually soup, bread followed by big slices of cream cheese, and an oily salad.

After supper the *evacués* – the men who got their new clothes and big boots in the afternoon – are to go up to the Hospice, the other hospital on the hill at the farther end of the village. The hoot of the car is heard as it comes round from the garage; the men are collected and squeeze into the ambulance; we dash up the street, and in two minutes are at the gates of the Hospice, where there are many old acquaintances among the wounded to greet us. The men pre allotted to their wards, and then we dash back with the car; for there are a couple of stretcher-cases also to be fetched. These are lifted in, and on arrival at the Hospice must be carried up to their beds.

At last I flatter myself that work is over for the day, and pass through the château for a stroll in the cool air of the park. But on my way I am seized by the Matron. There is a French bedstead to be got up from the cellar for an isolation case in the turret-room. Two of us depart on the errand. French bedsteads are not like ours. They fold up in the middle. They have sharp edges everywhere and crab-like propensities to pinch. They fold and unfold when you least expect it, and catch your flesh unawares. And what they catch they grip. Carrying one of these vindictive machines up three flights of stairs is a journey of pain. The bedstead kicks and pinches at every step. But at last it is got up into the room, and set up on its four feet, and a mattress thrown on it to keep it from further convulsions. We heave a sigh of joy, and leave a grateful Sister.

Now surely we have half an hour's peace before our own

supper. I find Sebastien, my Breton friend, under the tulip-tree, full of reproaches because I am so late for the promised stroll. And we are just starting when a shout from someone calls me back. What can it be? A hæmorrhage? I start to run at the thought. Blessed relief! It is only fourteen casks of wine which have arrived, and someone is wanted to roll them into the cellar. In the courtyard I find two high carts, each with a pair of horses harnessed tandem, and each loaded with barrels. How are the barrels to be got off the carts? Everything points to a stretcher; and finding an old stout English stretcher, I slant it from the cart-tail to the ground. The barrels come rolling down with a little counter-pressure to ease their descent; and before long the whole fourteen are rolled into place.

There is still time for a little ramble; and I saunter with Sebastien along the little river, where every now and then a trout rises and flops in the cool stillness of the twilight. Sebastien has lost a hand; but, as he tells me, '*J'ai toujours de la chance*': it might have been the right hand, and it is the left. Also, he had always hoped, if he were wounded, for two things: first to be taken to a château, and second, to be in an English hospital. *Et me voici!* He is a good soldier, but he does not like the war at all. He tells me all about his home at Quimper and his boyhood. He wants to come to England. I have been trying to teach him a little English, but the words he learns to pronounce with difficulty become more and more unrecognisable each time he repeats them. It is true, our pronunciation is formidable enough for a French tongue; and he is also rather lazy. His education is inconsiderable; but his manners are perfect in their natural ease and grace.

Having set down these common tasks which make up the

orderly's day, I feel half-ashamed at proffering so trivial a record, when the real work of the hospital, the work of the doctors and nurses, who have not only hard labours to perform with their trained skill, but endless anxious responsibilities, is the story that ought to be told. Alas, I have not the knowledge for the telling of it; I have only boundless honour and admiration for them and their wonderful work. We orderlies have glimpses only of what that work means, what lives it saves, what suffering it alleviates. We see rather the human side; yet that is my excuse for these pages, since I hope they may reflect something of the qualities of the Poilu whom we love, as we have learnt to know him in his hour of trial and suffering; gentle in speech, courteous in bearing, constant in fortitude, fervent in the faith of his country's cause.

THE CANTEENS

I

With the account of the Convoys and the Hospitals we conclude our record of the Red Cross work done by the British for the French wounded.

But there are other ways in which we have been able to help the French soldier.

Quite early in the war an organisation for providing canteens for the refreshment of the sick and tired soldiers was set on foot in Paris by a patriotic Frenchman.

It was called '*L'Œuvre de la Goutte de Café.*' It was on a small scale, on account of the limited funds available; but the first canteens which it started were so greatly appreciated and so obviously needed that the founder of the Œuvre and his wife, whose hearts were very much in the work, looked about for means to extend it.

One day the *Présidente* of the *Comité Britannique* received a letter asking if funds from England could be made available for establishing more canteens. *Madame la Présidente* had a great desire to further this work, if possible. And it occurred to her that the application might be turned to an even greater and more beneficent opportunity than had been originally contemplated. For every day the *Comité* was being approached by Englishwomen who wanted to serve France in some way, yet had no specific training or qualification. Here was at once an outlet for their enterprise and enthusiasm, and a golden occasion for furthering the friendship of the two countries. The application of the *Œuvre de la Goutte de Café* had been for funds; but how infinitely better to provide not only funds but personal service! How much more it would mean to the French soldier if he could see and grasp hands with these Englishwomen whose love for France prompted them to go out and do hard work for the comfort and refreshment of the Poilu, than if he were merely told that certain funds had been contributed by English people!

So it came to be arranged by mutual consent that the *Comité Britannique* should undertake the setting-up of additional canteens, and should provide their *personnel*.

Any one who has visited France during the war will have been forced at every turn to realise the great difference that the habit of military service makes to a nation. Every boy in France knows that, except in special circumstances, a period of service with the colours lies before him, and that for the best part of his life he will be liable to service. Every mother knows that her son is bound to pass through these years of training, and in case of war, is bound to fight. It is all part of the national life; it is all taken for granted.

But with us in England how different it was! Only a minute fraction of those now fighting ever dreamed for a moment of being a soldier. The vast majority had no interest in military matters whatever. Our millions of volunteers, when they enlisted, undertook something that was absolutely novel, and was a complete break with all their habits, interests, and traditions. It was like going out into an unknown country; an immense, life-absorbing adventure. And the rest of our population, that saw sons, brothers, husbands, and lovers go out into this terrible new world for the sake of their country's cause, how eagerly it followed them with its love and admiration; how it resolved to do everything possible for their comfort and support when they were not actually fighting in the -misery of the trenches; how it lavished generosity on the wounded! Organisations like the Y.M.C.A., and the Church Army devoted energies to building recreation huts and starting canteens for the soldiers behind the lines in France or at camps in England; and money poured in from the public for these purposes.

There are no such great organisations in France. There, the soldier takes his service as a matter of course, and the public takes it also as a matter of course. The men are doing what they have always been expected to do, in case of war arising; and the whole nation shares alike. The French soldier rubs along with little enough; his wants are easily satisfied, at least he puts up with what he gets, and is not given to complaining. His pay is five sous a day; and that is five times as much as he was given at the beginning of the war. And he has very little – scarcely any – of all that extra, non-official provision for his comfort that has been made for our soldiers.

But this war is unparalleled alike in its intensity and pro-traction. Men can face hardship and physical misery, and daily danger of death and wounds, with comparative cheer-fulness, if the end be in sight; if they know that misery, hardship, and danger are only for a certain term. But to endure for years without coming nearer to an end is a terrible exaction on the hardiest nerves. And when the pressure is lightened for a moment; when the men are resting, or travelling wearily to and fro from the lines; then is the time – the empty time – when they need to be refreshed and entertained, to have their thoughts diverted, above all to recover the touch of something human, something apart from the nations' rivalry of destruction. The canteens and the recreation huts are little islands of refuge in the ocean of waste and loss and monotonous hardship. More and more as the war drags on their value is appreciated. It was therefore a prescient patriotism which inspired *L'Œuvre de la Goutte de Café*. And we in Britain may well be glad that we have been able to help and so considerably to extend work of such living, tonic influence.

II

The canteens fall into four classes : those at Railway Stations, those at *Foyers de Cantonnement*, those at *Dépôts des Éclopés*, and those at *Dépôts d'Isolés*. These terms need some explanation.

A *Dépôt des Éclopés* is a military depot where tired but not wounded soldiers are sent for a few weeks' rest. The canteens attached to these may be asked to do some light cooking, or cooking of invalid dishes, for the worse cases in the sick ward.

A *Dépôt d'Isolés* is a military depot for men who are passing through on their way to be re-drafted to their regiment or re-equipped. They stay for one or two days; sometimes less, very rarely more.

A *Foyer* is a recreation-room where the men can sit and read, smoke, play games, and write letters.

Foyers are attached to rest camps to which an *armée au repos* is sent for a rest of more or less duration, the men being billeted in the villages chosen for their cantonments.

These various posts are started by the English 'canteeners' wherever possible.

Gramophones are an essential part of the equipment of a canteen. In many canteens the *Dames Anglaises* have set up a cinema, which is especially enjoyed during the long evenings of the winter months. Whenever it can be done, concerts and entertainments are got up.

At the canteens, refreshments such as coffee, soup, cocoa, biscuits, jam, sweets, and other dainties are served out. Except at the *Dépôts des Éclopés* there is no cooking of dishes. English cigarettes and tobacco are also distributed. Many of the French soldiers prefer them to what they get in France.

In all the canteens organised through the *Comité Britannique* everything is given free. In those worked by other societies, under the auspices of the *Comité*, a nominal charge is made.

The *Comité* sends out under-linen, socks, mufflers, gloves, handkerchiefs, etc., to be given to the soldiers when needed. A lady writes from one canteen, acknowledging a parcel of socks, that 'we often have to attend to sore feet, and we are glad of socks to give the men to change. We do quite a number of dressings in a small way, and we keep a good supply of dressings and all kinds of remedies for various ailments.'

The fact that things are given free, and that English ladies have come out of their own accord to do this hard work for the French, are two things that have greatly touched the *Poilus*. At first, indeed, their surprise at things so unexpected inclined them almost to think that some design upon them was intended. But if any such misgivings were entertained they soon vanished.

It was in February 1915 that the first of the *Comité*'s canteens was started, at Hazebrouck railway station. It was under an engagement to feed no English, but there were Belgians as well as French among those who frequented it.

'We started on 2nd February,' wrote the lady in charge in her first report, 'and up to last night, 24th February, we have fed 11,007 wounded, reinforcements and refugees. We have given them coffee, chocolate, milk, soup, bread, cigarettes, and papers. We find chocolate the most popular drink, and so make most of that. We make all the drinks strong and as nutritious as possible, the chocolate always having milk and sugar. We have the plain milk or tea for the fever cases, and milk for the refugee babies... I have built a hut in the stationmaster's garden for my canteen, and during the morning there are always five or six French soldiers in having their breakfast... I have two soldiers working for me, and they do all the heavy lifting and carrying; and two more come when the trains come in. We all enjoy the work and are very enthusiastic.'

This canteen was soon afterwards transferred to Doullens.

In this same spring four more canteens were started. One was attached to a *Dépôt d'Isolés* at Le Bourget, in the suburbs of Paris.

It was opened in March. About the same time, a canteen was opened in a *Dépôt des Éclopés* at Le Courneuve on the northern outskirts of Paris. Another at Creil was started in the railway station; a third at Crézancy for *Éclopés*, and a fourth at Doullens station, transferred from Hazebrouck. This last was closed in the spring of 1917.

In June, two canteens for *Éclopés* were opened; one at Drancy, in the northern outskirts of Paris, the other at Lure in the Haute Saône department, afterwards transferred to Remiremont in the Vosges. In August, three more canteens for *Éclopés*: at Le Tréport, Hesdin (closed in April 1916), and Puys (closed in June 1917). In September a canteen for *Éclopés* was started at Doullens, afterwards transferred to Poix; in October, one at Vaivre, afterwards transferred to Hericourt.

In November a canteen for Isoles was opened at St-Dizier in the Haute Marne; and one for *Éclopés* at Montataire, on the Oise, afterwards transferred to Villers-Cotterets, near Soissons.

December brought the second Christmas of the war, and the English workers in France made a point of celebrating it after the English fashion. We get a glimpse of how Christmas was kept at a canteen for Isoles from a letter written home from St-Dizier, on December 27th:

> We had a very nice day and evening on the 25th. Two hundred soldiers turned up, and when they saw the canteen all lit up they nearly went mad. We had two Christmas trees given us, and a man in the town had them all lit with electric light in coloured globes. Another shop lent us the little glistening things to put on, and we made paper flowers, so it looked very pretty, but we tried putting the small presents on the night before, and naturally during the night they were all stolen, so decided to only make the tree look nice and hand the presents round after supper. Only Miss W——'s parcels had arrived (mine have not turned up yet), so we had not really enough to go round and had to wait a bit till some of the men had to leave. We had sixteen tables lent us, also chairs, and, with white paper put on instead of tablecloths, they looked very clean. Madame B—— and her sister-in-law helped us, and we each took so many tables. Their menu was the following:

Hot soup.
Cold ham.
Hot roast beef and haricot beans
Bread and jam.
Red wine (a gift).
Coffee.
Cigars and cigarettes (gifts from Commandant de R. and Capt. B.).
After the feast we had songs and recitations and the gramophone (which Miss W—— bought in Paris; it goes all day long and they adore 'Tipperary.')
They then made speeches; most embarrassing. We were called up under the platform, and had the most charming things said to us. Also passionate love songs sung with much feeling right into our faces. We also had a book on the table and asked for their names. I enclose a few of the remarks written. I do not know if you can read them. The Arabs wrote their names back to front, and kept licking the pen, and instead of writing any remark put rows of xxxx... I felt fearfully happy that we had given so much joy to the poor French soldiers. They so love being waited on; or any little attention we show them they make much of. The town folk were awfully kind in giving us presents for the tree, and other money. Altogether we had three hundred francs given us to spend for them.

And how Christmas puddings were made and eaten – a great adventure for the *Poilus* – is told by the *Directrice* of another canteen:

The *Médecin-chef* has been persuaded to let us give plum-pudding *à l'anglaise* on Christmas Day to the men on the *petit régime,* and one evening towards the middle of December found us feverishly searching for the ingredients. Most of them we succeeded in getting through the *infirmier* who did the daily commissions, but treacle (which with sundry other unexpected items was enjoined in the old family recipe which we were following) was another matter. Our grocer was not only unable to produce it, but was astonished at being asked for it. 'You may find it at a druggist's,' she said doubtfully. However, we found it at last at another grocer's, where it is known as 'golden,'and the weights and scales required we were able to borrow from an umbrella shop. (This does not necessarily imply that in A. umbrellas are sold by weight, but all these preliminaries were a little suggestive of "Alice in Wonderland.")

Then came the great day of chopping and stoning and mincing and mixing, and every one at hand was called in to stir the mysterious mass. None of our friends, it seemed, had ever eaten English plum-pudding, but one boy maintained that he knew what it was like. It was 'something fried in oil' and he added loyally that his mother knew how to make it. Various little basins were filled for friends who were not likely to be with us on Christmas Day, and the remainder we tied up in a cloth so as to secure the orthodox globular form depicted on Christmas cards. Early in the morning they were put on to boil, but alas! in the course of the afternoon a catastrophe occurred which became painfully apparent when the puddings were taken up. The pudding had stuck to the bottom of the big *marmite* in which it was cooking, a hole had been burnt in the cloth, and through the hole the precious contents were oozing into the water. A considerable amount escaped, but it was not wasted, since a thrifty kitchen orderly put it into the soup. In the course of the struggle that ensued a chink was heard, and lo! a half-franc piece stood revealed, one of the exciting little objects which had been put in to give an added *éclat* to the pudding. '*Mais, Mademoiselle, c'est vous qui serez riche,*' exclaimed J., highly pleased; but we conscientiously restored the little coin through the hole whence it had issued before enveloping all in a fresh cloth, and not till that was done did the stone for poverty reveal itself.

In spite of all these vicissitudes the pudding made a brave show on Christmas Day, drenched in flaming brandy and crowned with a spray of holly. The guests were warned to investigate their helpings carefully, and not swallow such indigestible morsels as coins and rings, and the bachelor's button fell to a married man, to the great satisfaction of all the rest. Every crumb was finished, and presently we were waited upon by a deputation who made a very pretty speech of thanks.

But what, we wondered, of the little puddings which had gone to the trenches? Had their recipients managed to boil them, or eaten them cold and stodgy, yet not without a kindly thought of the canteen whence they came?

1916 was to see a great expansion of the work of the

canteens. In a good many cases, as will be seen, they were transferred to other posts, according to the need of the moment and the movement of the armies.

In January six canteens were opened. Two of these – one a station canteen, the other for *Éclopés* – were at Meaux. A station canteen was started at Crépy; a canteen for *Éclopés* at Quartier Songis, a military establishment in Troyes. A second canteen at Le Bourget was started this month, and in February a third was added, at the military exchange station connecting the Nord, Est, Lyons, and *ceinture* lines. Two canteens for *Éclopés* were started in February, one at Abbeville (closed in June 1917), the other at St-Amand-sur-Fion, afterwards transferred to Beauvoir.

In March a canteen for *Éclopés* was opened at Domremy, the birthplace of Joan of Arc. It was transferred later to Neuf chateau. In April two - canteens for *Éclopés* were opened : at Dainville, also transferred later to Neufchâteau; and at Rambervillers in the Vosges.

In May, four canteens were added to those in *Dépôts des Éclopés*. These were at Vertus, Bar-sur-Aube, St- Just, and Vendeuvre. The last was closed in January 1917.

In June a canteen for *Isolés* was opened at Arc-les-Gray.

In July two station canteens were started: one at Troyes, the other at Revigny, near Bar-le-Duc. A canteen for *Éclopés* was opened at Poix.

In August three canteens for *Éclopés* began work : at Conty, at Neufchâteau, and at Beauvoir.

In September, canteens for *Éclopés* were opened at Amiens (closed October 1917), Grandvillers (transferred later to La Ferté Milon), and Thury-en-Valois. A *Foyer* was opened at Triaucourt, another at Villers-Cotterets, and a station canteen was started at the same time at the latter place.

A canteen for *Isolés* was started at Besançon in October, transferred later to Arc-les-Gray.

In December a canteen for *Éclopés* was opened at Remiremont, in the Vosges.

In January 1917 a station canteen was started at Bussang, and one in March at Survilliers.

A canteen for *Éclopés* was opened in April at Toul; three more in May, at La Ferte Milon, Mesgrigny, and Vertus. In May also a *Foyer* was opened at Epernay, and a station canteen at Orry-la-Ville. A station canteen was added at Epernay a little later.

In June a canteen for *Éclopés* was opened at Allonne, afterwards transferred to Vasseny; and another at Herme, afterwards transferred to Méry-sur-Seine. In the same month a *Foyer*, as well as a canteen for Eclopes, was opened at Ay: both of these were transferred later, one to Avenay, the other to Braine. A canteen for *Isolés* was also started at Connantre.

In July a station canteen was opened at Jessains; a canteen for *Éclopés* at Antilly, another at Beugneux, and a *Foyer* at Avenay.

In August a station canteen was opened at Braine, and another at Oulchy-Brény. A *Foyer* was opened at Vasseny.

In September a canteen for *Éclopés* was started at Mery-sur-Seine, transferred later to Fére-en-Tardenois.

In October a *Foyer* was opened at Jubécourt, and station canteens at Corcieux, Mourmelon-le-Petit, and Wesserling.

In November six *Foyers* were opened: at Bucy-le-long, Bouvancourt, Courcelles, Fére-en-Tardenois, Pommiers, and Vitry-le-François.

At the moment of writing (December 1917) *Foyers* are in process of formation at the following places : Champigneul, Provins, St-Amand, St-Lumier.

III

Reference to the map will show that these canteens are almost all distributed on lines radiating from Paris to the front. As will be seen from the foregoing list, they have been steadily increasing in number, in response to an ever growing demand.

At first there was a certain hesitation on the part of some of the military authorities, due to anxiety lest the canteens should lead to relaxation of discipline. But no such result has followed, while the temper of the soldiers, war-weary as they are, has been fortified by the thought and care bestowed on them : it has put new courage into their hearts.

To show how the officers in command appreciate what the canteens do for their men, here is a letter from the Commandant d'Étapes at R. written on the 9th of July 1917:

Madame, – Il y a un an à pareille date, dans une minuscule et très inconfortable baraque vous versiez votre première tasse de café aux permissionnaires de passage à R. Depuis une Cantine agrandie et par vos soins décorée avec un goût parfait, des flots de café, de thé, de choco-lat, de bouillon, des cigarettes par centaines de mille, des cadeaux de toute sorte ont été distribués aux "poilus" de Verdun.

Je ne puis laisser passer cette date du 9 juillet, sans vous en témoigner toute ma gratitude.

Depuis un an, de jour comme de nuit, vous êtes sur

la brêche apportant à nos soldats un réconfort de tous les instants; et cette tâche si pénible vous l'avez accomplie avec un dévouement, avec un art si parfait, que votre œuvre éminemment utile en point de vue matériel est devenue une œuvre de haute portée morale.

La Cantine Anglaise de R., c'est la Cantine de l'Armée de Verdun. Pour ceux qui "montent" c'est là qu'ils respirent les dernières effluves d'une sympathie si chaude qu'elle galvanise les cœurs les plus angoissés; pour ceux qui «descendent» couverts encore des boues de la tranchée, brisés des emotions de la lutte, c'est le premier sourire au seuil d'une vie que beaucoup ne comptaient plus revoir.

Aussi je n'hésite pas a le proclamer bien haut, vous êtes la providence de l'armée de Verdun.

Veuillez agréer, Madame, avec l'assurance de mon respectueux dévouement, l'expression de ma bien vive reconnaissance.

(Signature) Commandant B.,
Commandant d'Étapes de R.'

And to show how the soldiers keep up cordial relations with their English friends of the canteen, let me quote some sentences from a letter addressed to one of them by a Zouave who, after being at the *Dépôt*, had been wounded and lost a finger, and then sent to work as a miner. As he had had three years of the trenches, he was not ill-content. He begins: '*Ma chére Maman*,' and after telling of his wound and his work, goes on (I retain grammar and spelling):

Je tiend à vous mettre en mémoir que je suis le Zouaves en cas ou vous ne seriez plus qui je suis, et aujourd'hui j'ai reçue votre colis de cigarettes qui me fait un grand plaisir, je vous assure que voilà un moment qu'il voyage ce colis, mais tous est encore intacte. Je vous dirais que je n'est encore pas de nouvelles de mais Pauvre Parents resté à Lens. Je crois ma chère Maman que cette fois je suis Orphelin, me voilà complèment seul sur terre, ces pourquoi j'exprime l'exprestion en vous appelant Maman, je crois que cela ne vous dérangeras pas...

Again a *Directrice* reports:

All our relations with the men were of the most delightful character. Their gratitude was most touching, and the many letters we still receive show that 'out of sight is not out of mind' with them. Their extreme gratitude often made one feel quite humble that the very little we could do was magnified into such a big thing in their eyes.

And now, what does the actual work of the *Dames Anglaises* consist of?

Those who have had the pleasure of reading Mrs. Dixon's book – *The Canteeners*, published in 1917 – will have gained a vivid impression of daily life in canteens at Troyes, at Hericourt in the Vosges, and at the busy military station in the dingy Paris suburb of Le Bourget. But even those who have read Mrs. Dixon's little volume may like to hear something further of this work of their countrywomen; and we will add here brief accounts given by the workers themselves of a day at a canteen at a *Dépôt d'Isolés*, a day at a canteen in a *Dépôt des Éclopés*, and a day at a *Foyer* in a rest camp:

At a Cantine d'Isolés

About 8.30 one of us arrives at the canteen. Tables and chairs outside washed and dusted over. Games put out and the inkstands and writing things. Tisane made in the large *marmite*, which holds about 500 cups. This lasts two days as a rule – and is warmed up the second day, as they like it hot. It is extremely simple to make, being only *bois de réglisse* tied in a muslin bag and put into a large urn of boiling water and a few handfuls of mint or camomile, in another small piece of muslin, put in to flavour it. The men stand outside the hut, and they help themselves as they like. About 10.30 the other ladies arrive and then we make the coffee, the water for which is already boiling, and fires kept up by our own orderly, who also washes out the hut for us and fetches water and lights all the fires before we come. He also cleans the chimneys three times a week, which is *most* necessary to make them burn.

The coffee is ready by 11.30 and distributed at the window of the canteen, two of us usually pouring out, one giving a sheet of paper and an envelope to every one who wishes for it, and on Wednesdays and Sundays they get a cigarette each also.

This is the chief feature of the day, and gives great pleasure, as the dejeuner is at 11, and the hot coffee after it is much appreciated. We generally have our own combined tea and luncheon about 2.20, and tidy up the hut, as it is a very dirty and smoky place.

At 1.30 we take a small jug of milk food to the infirmaries who care for it, especially the men who cannot eat solid food, generally Benger's food, or crême d'orge, and one can take them any little present or comforts also; slippers are very useful, and we have had a gift of 25 pairs from the Belgravia War Work Rooms.

There are four infirmaries, generally full, but as a rule no serious cases or wounds are sent there, only minor illnesses and wounds, frostbitten feet, sprains, etc.

At 2.30 we have another distribution of cocoa (which is called chocolate), and this too is generally liked.

About every other day there is a departure for the front of 10 to 50 men, and they generally let us know, when we give them a few cigarettes (3 to 5) and a small souvenir – a small looking-glass is a very favourite one, and also pencils, writing-cases, which can be got at home for 5d. now, and they also greatly like cards of London (6 for a 1d. at Straker's, 3 or 4 series of them.) The gramophone is a great pleasure, and we think of leaving it here. There are some good records. English songs are not much use, we find, but good French songs or opera selections, flute or cornet solos, etc., are very suitable and give much pleasure; they like them very much in the infirmaries too, and it is often borrowed for an hour or so. One very favourite amusement is zigzag puzzles – of which one cannot have too many. Also cards; and we have introduced 'Halma,' also 'Spoof,' with good effect. A small board with India rubber rings and darts to throw at a cardboard target; bumble-puppy, played with old lawntennis racquets, now mostly broken, etc., are all popular. We have also attempted Clock

Golf. They love talking too – of their wives and families – as they are not allowed to go out at all, and their families, even if quite near, only allowed to come for an hour in the afternoon; they feel like prisoners. Sometimes one can do messages and commissions for them, getting a watch repaired, buying something or other – and many little odds and ends. We were able to let one man's wife know where he was, to their pleasure, as they are not allowed to mention the name of the place in writing. They seem quite to look upon us as friends, and certainly the canteen helps to brighten them and make what would be a very dreary time of convalescence and repose into a bright and cheery one, and we get many letters and postcards from them when they leave, thanking us for what we have done.

At 5 o'clock they have soup, and the day is over. We therefore catch the 5 o'clock train back to Paris – in a quarter of an hour. This makes an excellent starting point.'

At a Cantine des Éclopés

It is 9am, and the first lady on duty arrives. She hopes (and is not usually disappointed, as the orderly is a very efficient one) to find the big *marmite* coming to the boil on its *réchaud*. The said orderly, who claims descent from St. Louis, has probably been there since 6.30am cleaning up, carrying the water for the day and lighting the fires. There are two *réchaud*s and two stoves in the small canteen kitchen, although usually the *réchaud*s and the large stove are sufficient. On this stove is another *marmite*, only smaller, in which the morning's bouillon and puree are cooking. Bouillon and puree de legumes, which seem essentially French fare, are very simple in their making. Any available vegetables (and when are masses of vegetables not available in France, even in war-time, though at war-prices – particularly where English purses are concerned?) – carrots, turnips, potatoes, cabbage, etc., are all sliced up and boiled in the big pot. The vegetables are then fished out from the bouillon, and passed through a cullender until, as a delightful squash and mixed with some white sauce, they are served out in portions to those men in the infirmary who are on special diet, and to the *édentés*, the dentist's patients whose toothless condition is supposed to render them unable to eat the barrack ration, but who we strongly suspect often manage to consume the two!

A liberal allowance of sugar and the bags of coffee having now been put into the big *marmite* and a few odd jobs done, such as arranging flowers round the statuette of Joan of Arc and putting out illustrated papers and puzzles (the men love 'Jig-Saws', and the ‹Road to Serbia' and 'French Football' are always wearing out owing to constant use and vigorous shakings) on the trestle table in front of the canteen, where benches are also provided, we are ready for the chief business of the day – the serving out of the coffee. The stream of customers begins about 10.30, when the bugle sounds the first '*Soupe*' – the *déjeuner a la fourchette* of the *Ésclopés* – these are the men sent into the barracks for minor ailments.

The first to come are orderlies from the infirmary

and the *édentés* to fetch the bouillon and purée, and any still more special diets that they may have been ordered by the *Médecin-chef*, such as eggs, or a portion of beef-steak, or purée of macaroni, which is often given in place of the purée of légumes.

There are messengers with pails and armed with *bons* signed by the sergeant of each bâtiment, to say how many are to have coffee sent to them. These *bons* are always rather mysterious; for all the men in these barracks except those in the infirmary are supposed to be walking cases, but many, sometimes to the number of fifty or sixty in a bâtiment, seem to prefer their morning coffee taken to them, and this number has an amusing way of increasing if the day happens to be wet.

After the pails are disposed of, our regular customers arrive, those who having finished their meal like to stroll round to the canteen and have a little chat over their morning cup, or *'quart'* of coffee. These *'quarts'* (quarter of a litre measure) are typically French, a tin cup which every soldier carries in his pocket, or hidden somewhere about his uniform, and one cannot help thinking what an immense saving of labour it would make in the strenuous 'washing up' in some of our English canteens, if our men did the same! But perhaps the British Tommy would hardly appreciate the one tin cup to serve all purposes when he is not actually in the trenches; and certainly these quarts show few signs of any washing between the various drinks – red wine, coffee, tea, lemonade, cocoa – which are poured into them.

It is now about 11.30, and the three lady workers,

for the other two have now arrived, sit down to a hurried lunch before the next stream, which has "soupe," somewhat later commences. These are the '*Petits Blessés,*' and form a long procession, as their bâtiments send no pails. These barracks were intended for *Éclopés* only, but during the big offensive in Champagne this spring and summer, half of them were given over to the '*Petits Blessés,*' and very glad we were to take them on among our customers. They are a wonderfully cheery, patient, and amusing crowd, and very ready to talk and recount their experiences; but at this hour there is little time except to say '*bonjour,*' and to hear if there is any special news, for by now the morning papers have arrived, and if the English have made any especially brilliant bit of advance, they are here to be the first to tell us. It takes two workers all their time, one pouring out through the canteen window, and the other filling the pipes from the big *marmite* behind, to get the stream passed along.

When that is over a jug of coffee is taken down to the Ambulance Infirmary for those who are too wounded to walk, and also picture papers, books, puzzles, and writing paper – for the French Poilu is a great scribe and his wife too; a man will often say how anxious he is if he has not had a letter from home for three days!

From 1 to 2.30 there is rather a pause, as the men are having their afternoon rest, and the early worker goes home while the other two write French letters and make up packets of cigarettes for the men who have gone back to the trenches. This keeping in touch with our old customers is one of the delightful parts of canteen work, and the men write such charming letters. The French Poilu is much less reserved than our English Tommy; he does not try to hide his feelings, and loves to talk about his wife and children or his fiancee, and to tell of the doings of his regiment. It is not that our Tommies are less patriotic in their attitude towards the war, but that the Frenchman does not mind expressing what he feels, particularly in his letters.

Many of the men give us their addresses when they leave, and some who have no relations ask us to become a Marraine (Godmother) for the war, as they do appreciate having someone to write to and who will write to them.

But to return to the daily routine of the Cantine. During the afternoon lemonade is served out, or, if it should be cold, tea or coffee, which the men are very fond of. Unless it is wet, the gramophone is brought out, and the men sit on the benches in front of the canteen, smoking (for cigarettes are handed round) and looking at the papers. They are very fond of the gramophone, and sing the French songs, especially those from well-known operas, best of all – often though they will ask for English songs, 'Tipperary' or 'Rule Britannia,' though one always has a suspicion that this is due to French politeness and out of compliment to us. They have a great admiration for the English soldiers, and will always tell us with great pride if they have been beside any of our troops, and if they have made friends with them or exchanged presents. The English hospitals, too, seem to amaze and delight them. The nursing, the splendid food, the jam, the luxuriousness of it all, impresses them very much. Several had been in English hospitals at Havre or along the coast, and one man, who had been at the Scottish Women's Hospital at Royaumont, was very full of the happy time he had spent there. At 5 p.m. more bouillon and puree and special diets are sent out to the infirmary, and at 6 p.m. the canteen closes.

There are certain variations in the work. One afternoon a week we give a gramophone concert in the Ambulance Infirmary, also serving '*dessert*,' stewed fruit and custard, to those who are not able to come to the canteen. These 'Smoking Concerts' are very popular.

Two days a week '*partants*' leave; those men returning to the front, and this forms quite a little ceremony. We are warned of the number beforehand, and then when the men are fully equipped in their new uniforms, with all their paraphernalia (including always a large loaf of bread and one or two tins of *Singe* (bully beef) strapped on their backs, they come to the canteen to say '*Au Revoir*.' They always insist on this form of good-bye, though they can only return by being ill or wounded! Each man carries away some packets of cigarettes, a slab of chocolate, writing-paper, a very gaudy red handkerchief "made in Birmingham," which they seem to prize greatly, and a *porte-bonheur*, a little medal of the Virgin or one of the Saints.

Sunday is a great morning in the barracks, the authorities providing an extra good *soupe*, often adding asparagus or some luxury that may be plentiful, and each man gets three cigarettes from us when he comes for his coffee. To arrange this fairly and to prevent overlapping, we devised a system of counters which much amuses the men. On Saturday the two bureaux, those of the *Éclopés* and the Ambulance, obtain from us the number of counters they require and distribute them, and on Sunday morning each man returns his counter to the canteen and gets his three cigarettes.

About once a month and on special fête-days we present cigarettes to the Guard and also to the Chasseurs, the large body of men who are employed in looking after the sick and wounded horses, for the outer ring of the barracks contains stabling for hundreds of horses sent down from the front to be cured or otherwise disposed of.

The distribution of cigarettes amounts to about twelve thousand a month, and is the largest item of the canteen expenses, as in our barracks the authorities allow us to "toucher" the coffee and sugar.

Once a week the authorities provide a concert in the barracks, which, if fine, is held out of doors. These concerts are often very good indeed, though the artistes are nearly all from among the men themselves, but in a Republican Conscript Army there are naturally all sorts and conditions of men and of talent.

A description of the canteen would be incomplete without mention of the Arabs and Senegalese – for we have many of these. The Algerian Arabs are generally very delightful and appreciative, and very happy when one can talk to them about their own country. They seem rather in banishment, as, when their '*Permission*' comes, they are not allowed to go home, possibly owing to the dangers of the crossing and also to the time it would take out of the eight days allowed, but are sent to some place in France, which though no doubt very pleasant is hardly the same as their beloved Algeria.

They especially appreciate our coffee, as most of them keep strictly to their religion and never drink the wine which is served out in the barrack rations. On the whole, though, they seem fairly content, as they mix happily with the other men, and generally speak French fairly well. Coming, too, from a warlike race, they do not seem to dislike their job, and love to tell of the fighting in which they have taken part – their description of how the Arab fights, taking no prisoners, being sometimes a little too graphic.

The most pathetic men are the Senegalese, as they understand very little French and seem to be like little children, drawn into a vortex which they do not understand. Like children though, they are made happy by very small things – they love sweets, and it is amusing to see a huge Senegalese beaming with joy over a handful of peppermints (their chief favourites) or an extra allowance of sugar in the pail of coffee that he has been sent to fetch for his *bâtiment*!

At a Foyer du Soldat

It is nine o'clock and we are opening for the day. Already there waits a crowd of shivering *Poilus* very eager for the hot coffee which is ready in a huge *marmite*, which will be filled again and again before the end of the day. A bowl of coffee and a crust of bread content the abstemious Frenchman, and he soon goes off to the duties of the morning, or, if *au repos*, settles down to his newspaper or a game of draughts or chess. In come some *'passage'* men in full marching kit, who demand bouillon, and are glad to lay aside their heavy packs and sit down and rest while it is being prepared. The next arrivals are half a dozen Moroccans, brownfaced and turbaned; sometimes we have Senegalese with jet-black skin and dazzling white teeth, or sallow Mongolians from Cochin; or perhaps a party of Breton *permissionnaires*, with an hour or two to wait between trains, comes in to while away the time with a game of cards or *'jacquet.'* And presently every one is at the windows to watch a battalion swinging down the street on its way to the trenches – a symphony of soft dull blue in the wintry sunshine, from helmet to puttees – all that *bleu horizon* which will presently melt into the blue mists lying in the forest glades, and so be lost to sight. Very gay and cheery they are, from the band which leads to the humble field-kitchens which bring up the rear, but we notice some wistful glances directed to the *Foyer* windows. But they may not stop; we can only wave our hands and wish them *'bonne chance,'* and on they go, while we return to the interrupted coffee making and the other duties of a busy morning.

At noon we close the large room for a couple of hours, so that it may be swept and aired in readiness for the afternoon, and one worker remains to make chocolate for the evening, while the others go off to lunch. From one to two there is an English lesson, at which six or seven pupils of varying degrees of proficiency present themselves. They are very keen to learn, and enjoy the lessons as much, we hope, as their teachers, in spite of the difficulties of the terrible English 'th' and the vagaries of our pronunciation, so trying to the logical French mind.

Before we are ready for it, two o'clock has struck and the business of the afternoon begins. The room is fuller now than in the morning; more coffee is asked for, and between four and five, when hot and thirsty footballers come in and demand tea – often in very good English – you might almost fancy yourself in a YMCA hut. But there is no sale of tickets here – no payment of any kind, for everything is given free. We are under the auspices of the British Committee of the French Red Cross, and, as is the rule in all their canteens, nothing may be charged for. The French private soldier's pay is still only 2d. a day, unless he is actually in the trenches, and, though some have means of their own, others, men from the *pays envahi* are terribly poor.

From five o'clock onwards the room grows fuller and fuller, and by the time every one has come back from *la soupe* (the evening meal) every table is occupied, many games are going on, and a hefty pianist is playing rag-time on the long-suffering piano, to a circle of admiring friends.

The red *chechias* of a little party of Zouaves strike a bright note of colour at a table near the counter. One of the quartette is rather excited, and remarks '*Madame, je vous aime,*' to the lady who has just handed him a bowl of coffee. His friends, scandalised, explain, '*Il a trop bu,*' which, alas, is pretty obvious. But drunkenness is very rare, and we hardly ever have to turn out an obstreperous client. It is very difficult to enforce a rule which forbids our guests to stand on benches, chairs, and tables, for when the music begins – and there is generally more or less of a concert going on between 6.30 and 8 – there simply is not standing room on the floor. But the inevitable crowding and jostling is taken in good part, and anything like quarrelling is unknown.

The music is, naturally, of varying quality. Sometimes we have a singer or violinist who is known in the concert-rooms of Paris or Nice; sometimes the performer is a shy boy who forgets his words and is not very sure of the tune, but always the audience listens with enjoyment; faces are turned expectantly towards the piano, and the demand for coffee slackens for a while.

At a quarter to eight, it is time to begin the giving out of chocolate – a beverage which is very, very popular.

Bowls are filled and emptied, washed and refilled again and again, till perhaps two hundred have been given out, and a warning whistle from the corporal in charge tells us that it is time to close. Some of our friends leave 'wi' deefficulty,' but we have to be firm, for the cafes in the town are obliged to shut at eight, and rules are rules. A good deal of clearing up has to be done, and chocolate provided for the excellent helpers who have worked hard for us all the evening; but all is finished by 8.30; our good friend the corporal unbolts the big door – carefully barred to prevent the re-entering of strayed revellers – and sees us out with a cheery '*à demain.*'

There is little to mark the days – except the cigarettes which are given on Sundays and Thursdays – the excitement when a new division arrives, the lamentations when our best friends bid us goodbye and go back to the line.

Sunday is perhaps our busiest day, for that afternoon we have visitors from all the neighbouring villages. Four hundred bowls of coffee between two o'clock and *soupe* is no unusual amount to give, and the housekeeper has anxious moments, wondering whether enough coffee has been made, and if the sugar will hold out. We often use twenty pounds a day of the latter, and it is only to be had once in four days from the military authorities – needless to say, it is useless to ask for it at the shops.

Then there are days of bitter black frost, when there is no water or gas available, and we have to keep our friends waiting while the pipes are being laboriously thawed; wintry days when snow from two or three hundred pairs of feet covers the floor with slush; and mild days when we gasp for air, and are thankful when a newly broken window admits a welcome '*courant d'air.*'

If space permitted, and I were not afraid of wearying you, there are other things that I should like to tell you of – the Arts and Crafts Exhibition at Christmas, which evoked, besides the metal work in which the Poilu is proficient, sketches in oil and water-colour, embroidery (done in the trenches), poetry of no mean order, and musical compositions

– of the welcome given to our countrymen when one day some English artillery passed through the town, and 'Tipperary,' which is regarded as '*l'hymne anglaise*,' equally with 'God Save the King,' was called for and sung with acclamation. And I should like to quote from some of the letters which reach us, from camp and trench and dug-out, where amid hardships and danger and death men think gratefully of the peace and comfort of the *Foyer*. In graceful French or the quaintest of halting English, all are alike in their gratitude and affectionate appreciation of English friendship and goodwill...

Ever since January 1915 an independent society, the Women's Emergency Canteens, has maintained canteens and recreation-rooms at Compiègne and in various villages in that district, doing the most admirable work. A big barn will be taken for a *foyer*, and its bare interior transformed with the help of pictures, flags, and flowers. Across the farmyard will be the canteen, all spotless, where the steaming coffee is dispensed; while the English women-workers live in some small, deserted cottage near by – cold and uncomfortable, sometimes even dangerous, quarters. A portable cinematograph is part of the outfit of these canteens, and is a never-failing solace. The society has motor ambulances also, and conveys the sick and wounded from barge to hospital. But perhaps the best known part of its work is the canteens which it maintains in Paris. These are at the Gare du Nord and the Gare de Lyon. The former of these was opened in April 1915. It is in the basement of the station, and is open night and day. At six in the morning there are often two hundred men at breakfast. There is a hot dinner in the middle of the day, and on an average well over a thousand meals are served daily. Socks and shirts are provided, also writing-paper. There are beds for about sixty men, and recently a large dormitory has been added. The canteen at the Gare de Lyon is on a smaller scale. These canteens, where a small charge is made, are visited not only by the French, but by the British and all Allied soldiers.

A more recent independent enterprise is the Hackett-Lowther Unit, whose convoy service has been mentioned in the chapters on the convoys. Founded in August 1917, this unit is attached to certain sectors of the French front, and started its first canteen, recreation-room, and theatre in a big wooden hut not far from St-Quentin, in a village destroyed by the Germans on their retreat. The regiments supply performers for the concerts and entertainments given at the canteen, and there is no lack of distinguished talent; many of the performers are famous in the theatres of Paris. From three hundred and fifty to five hundred soldiers come every night from their damp and gloomy billets to the glow and animation, the cheering warmth and the music of the canteen.

RELIEF WORK
IN THE DEVASTATED ZONES

This chapter will chiefly be concerned with the labours of the Society of Friends.

During and after the Franco-Prussian War of 1870, there were several members of that society in England, who went out to do what they could for the civilian victims of the war. One or two of these recorded their experiences, which are of poignant interest to-day.

Following this example, members of the society formed, at the beginning of the present war, a War Victims Relief Committee. The activities of this body are quite distinct from that of the Friends' Ambulance Unit, the other Quaker organisation, of whose ambulance work we have already given some description. This Relief Committee has centres in Holland (for Belgian refugees), and in Russia, as well as in France; and also supplies workers for the Serbian Relief Committee. In each country there is a 'Field Committee' at headquarters, and local subcommittees at various places, directing the work in the several districts. Here, of course, it is of France only that we are to speak.

In the early autumn of 1914, the Relief Committee began its work in France. Its Field Committee sits in Paris. The area allotted by the Government for its labours was in the Departments of the Marne and the Meuse, a stretch of about sixty miles of country between Esternay and Bar-le-Duc. In the first month or two it had some thirty odd workers busy in the district; but by the following autumn these had been increased by about a hundred.

The expenditure has been between nineteen and twenty

thousand pounds a year.

The work done falls into four main categories – building; medical; distribution of clothing, furniture, etc.; and agriculture.

But above and beyond any material benefit, it was the aim of this committee, and of those who worked for it, to bring human sympathy, love, and consideration to the innocent sufferers stricken by the immense calamity of war. They were inspired by the motives which founded the Society of Friends; and as true Friends they have been recognised by those they laboured to help and reassure. While the efforts of the French nation in their supreme struggle were inevitably concentrated on the army defending their country's existence, and on the wounded, there seemed a special call to help the wives and children of the soldiers. And how vast a field of labour was opened up! Already after the battles of the Marne there were large tracts of Eastern France laid in ruins, and the inhabitants, either refugees or clinging in tenacious attachment to old homes, herded in the most miserable of shelters. A yet greater tract was, and still is, under German occupation. There the able-bodied men, husbands, fathers, and sons, had gone at once to their regiments; they are fighting or have been killed. Of the rest of the population, thousands are prisoners in Germany, thousands more are homeless. Those who have read *La Ville Envahie* know what kind of lot is theirs who stayed at home in the industrial towns of the north-east, subjected to a daily persecution as gross as it is mean and stupid, and inhumanly cut off from all communication, not only with their own kin and friends, but all the outer world. What a world of separation and heart-breaking on both sides of the barrier! How many families suddenly and horribly divided, ignorant whether those dearest to them are alive or dead, or where they are!

A number of French societies have dedicated themselves to the task of relieving this great welter of human misery; and with some of them the Friends' Committee have worked in close co-operation. In the beginning, the society was attached to the *Association des Infirmiére Visiteuses de France.* It was placed under the direct control of the *Service de Santé* and accredited by the *Service de Santé* to the *Préfets* of the Departments of Marne and Meuse. The *Préfets* gave the society a cordial welcome, and have expressed their gratitude in touching terms.

Any one who has seen the devastation wrought in the battles of the first autumn of the war, and through the deliberate burnings of villages carried out by the Germans, can imagine the utter prostration of mind in the homeless peasantry, used to their habitual peaceful toil, and in a day or a night violently thrown out of all that was the world to them into an unrecognised chaos and terrifying desolation. Without resources, knowing none but their neighbours and companions in ruin, they were stupefied by the shock; they did not know how to carry on an existence that held no future.

It was to combat this apathy of hopelessness, to reassure this despair, to revive the energy of life and will to work, that the Friends first addressed their efforts in the November of 1914.

The first thing to be done was to build huts and shelters for the homeless people who still remained in the devastated regions, miserably collected in cellars and outhouses. By that time great numbers of refugees had been sent down south and west into the interior; but thousands remained, either because they would not leave their old homes and the neighbourhood where their men were fighting, or because they had families of small children, or because of the congestion of the railways. Setting to work in their allotted district, the party of English helpers began to build wooden huts on a uniform plan. In time four hundred of these, with twenty-seven stables, were distributed among twenty-five villages, and accommodated thirteen hundred people. Thirty-six brick-and-timber houses accommodated ninety-six persons. The houses were built among the ruins of Sermaize, a little watering-place, in which the destruction has been signally complete. The material for these erections was supplied by the Departments concerned. With the building went an improved sanitation; a vital matter, as may be imagined, where everything was reduced to chaos, and none of the destitute inhabitants was capable of the physical and moral effort of attempting to restore the shattered mechanism of existence. The magnitude of the task might well have paralysed even the happy, strong, and healthy.

The next things to be provided were beds, bedding, furniture, kitchen utensils, and clothing. Beds and furniture were given to all whose houses had been burnt. But here a difficulty presented itself. The local records had all perished. Families had been separated, or had been lost; it was hard to identify them when found. In these circumstances, the only course was to decide each case on its merits. The cost of beds and furniture was shared by the Department and the Friends, or the French *Société du Bon Gîte*, and they were distributed by the committee.

By such prompt and effective measures the winter of 1914 was got through in supportable conditions.

With the spring of 1915 came the necessity of tilling and sowing the land. The able-bodied were all absent with the armies; those that were left had no heart to begin. But the presence of cheerful people ready to lend a hand, to give their companionship and sympathy, was persuasion that could not in the end be resisted. Seeds were given, and farming tools; stables and barns were rebuilt; threshing-machines were moved about the district, with skilled men to work them.

A great change has come over this ruined region, since the fire and ravage of the war swept over it. Earth has given her flowers; and, fortified and stimulated by help from willing workers, the forlorn *sinistrés*, as the burnt-out inhabitants are called, have made their improvised colonies among the mournful ruins into something resembling a home, and in their little houses and gardens have taken up once more the threads of a changed existence.

Earth has given her flowers; she has also given her weeds. And with the extreme scarcity of labour these have thriven and multiplied apace. It will take years to root them out from the vantage they have gained. In spite of heroic effort the condition of the land goes backward. That is, alas, inevitable!

The continuance of the war has not lessened the importance of this agricultural relief. The farmers have continued to receive help in the summer by the loan of implements and machines, in some cases worked by Friends. In the winter threshing is done on an increasingly large scale : in many villages the whole crop has been threshed by the English workers. A motor-tractor has been of great service in the Sermaize district, ploughing for the small farmers. Machines have been repaired in villages where the blacksmiths had been mobilised. Chickens and rabbits have been given away; and the distribution of seeds, on an even larger scale, has been extremely successful.

On the other hand, the distribution of clothing in the Marne district has now ceased, except for newly returned families.

By comparison with those who have remained on the soil, the lot of the emigres or refugees has become, as the war persists, far more to be pitied.

The two urgent problems are those of employment and of housing. Few of the refugees are able-bodied men : these can count on getting work. For the others employment is difficult to obtain, and at the best is apt to be intermittent and insecure. In the country women can find work on the farms for part of the year, and occasionally wash and cook for passing troops : in the towns they get tailoring and washing to do, and in some places munition-making. But when they are old and ailing, or kept at home by a mother's duties to small children, life is hard indeed. The Government allowance, with the cost of everything continually rising, is not sufficient without some earnings to supplement it; and the families who are prevented by their circumstances from supplementing the allowance suffer seriously from inadequate nourishment. As a measure of relief potatoes have been sold at cheap rates to refugees in villages where the crop has been poor or the supply precarious, since potatoes and bread are the staple food, and if these fail the conditions of the village is disastrous.

The situation is made worse by the difficulties of housing. It is hard to find lodgings in the towns, where exorbitant prices are charged for wretched quarters, and the refugees are crowded into slum tenements with disastrous results upon their health. At Troyes, for instance, where the Friends have a centre, there are some seven thousand refugees and quite inadequate accommodation. In Paris there are, or were, a hundred thousand. The committee has done its utmost with the funds available to better the lot of these refugees by schemes for providing them with employment, and also for housing them, as far as this is possible.

As part of the schemes for providing employment, sewing and embroidery classes have been set on foot at Bar-le-Duc, Châlons, and around Sermaize and Vitry. At Troyes, pillows and quilts are made, and sewing-machines lent or given.

Materials are supplied by the Friends. This has proved an excellent solace and distraction from the benumbing weight of grief. The women and girls thus employed speak of the scheme with real gratitude, and there is great eagerness to join in it. A mother told how she had heard her daughters, as they sat over their new-found occupation, singing for the first time since the war began. And a child of seven confided gravely: '*Pour les émigrés, vous savez, c'est désolant, mais avec la broderie, on s'ennuiera moins.*'

At Bar-le-Duc, where early in 1916 the refugees came streaming in from Verdun and its neighbourhood, there is a work-room where eighty women and girls are employed; and for over a hundred more, occupation has been found in various kinds of needlework, and in the fine white embroidery which many of them practised before the war. There is also a 'Linen Chest Club,' which has been an extraordinary success. A refugee family pays fr.1.50, and provides a packing-case. They receive three or four sheets, four pillow-cases, six towels, and a blanket, and are encouraged to embroider their initials on the linen. A carpenter adds clasps and hinges to the case, which thus becomes a small family linen-chest for the future. Nearly seven hundred families have been so provided.

The problem of housing is immense. Such part of it as the Friends' Committee has been able to deal with has been met in the main by a scheme for building portable houses.

At Dôle, in the Jura, there is a construction camp where these houses are made in sections. This work has greatly increased during the past year, and machinery has been installed which has made a far larger and more rapid production possible. A similar camp and workshops have also recently been opened at Ornans, near Besançon. The portable houses were intended for use in destroyed villages which an advance of the Allies would liberate from German occupation; and in the meantime it was proposed to house in them refugees who were living in wretched conditions in towns like Troyes, Châlons, and Paris. The advance in Picardy in the spring of 1917 brought a request for these houses from the Minister of the Interior; and a number already finished and destined for other districts were sent to the newly liberated region. Later on, others were substituted for them.

Here may be noted a contrast between the district devastated by the Marne battles and that which the Germans occupied and retreated from last year. Battle and burning had indeed left widespread damage and destruction in the wake of the German retreat in 1914; but in the area of the Somme and the Aisne, where the Friends are now working, the havoc has been far more uniformly systematic. A hundred and fifty villages have been destroyed in that area, a few by shell-fire, most by deliberate destruction.

Often it is found that every house, and even the church, has been blown up by dynamite. In this devastated region, the Friends are engaged on a large scheme of rebuilding, and, where the damage is not irretrievable, of repairing.

The opening up of new areas by the advance of the Allied Armies has made urgent claims on some of the housing material, which was first to have been used for refugees in the interior. None the less, energetic efforts have been made to procure the refugees better house-room; at Troyes, for instance, where the crowding is so serious a problem. These efforts are furthered by a system of buying furniture and selling it to the *émigrés* under cost price. The payments are made in the form of monthly hire. This system works well, and answers a very real need. For instance, it was found that one family of four had paid since the beginning of the war some 600 francs in rent for a tiny furnished attic. They had paid all this, yet owned nothing in the end. Had there been at the beginning such a system as the Friends had established, they could have rented an unfurnished room, and, buying furniture by instalments, they would have owned enough to start life again with, on their return to their homes.

Be it recorded to the honour of these poor and exiled French people that the sales to them of furniture and other goods have hardly resulted in any bad debts. They often pay the whole sum with astonishing rapidity.

But of all the problems now confronting those who set out to relieve the victims of the war, the greatest has come to be that of ill-health and disease. At first it was naked want and homeless misery that seemed the greatest evils. But with the gradual alteration of material condition, the more subtle and less visible effects of the great catastrophe begin to come to the surface. First, exposure and privation, then unhealthy housing, crowding together, and under-feeding have done their work; and the reaction of mind upon body, the passionate grief, the prolonged strain and isolation, the hope so long deferred, the gnawing anxieties of providing for the day's wants, have all combined to sap an enfeebled vitality. Now, in the fourth year of the war, the spread of disease, especially of tuberculosis, has become a terrible thing.

And this leads us to give some account of the medical side of the work of the Friends' Committee.

To go back to the beginning. When the pioneers of their expedition reached France in November 1914, a centre for medical work was started at Châlons-sur-Marne. The town itself had suffered little, for the Germans had only occupied it for nine days; but all around was the devastated district, filled with homeless folk who for one reason or another could not leave their villages. When the Friends made their offer of help to the Préfet of the Marne, his first thought was for the coming generation, and for the mothers expecting children; and he arranged for a maternity hospital in Châlons, to be installed in a block of buildings used as a home for old people of the Department who could not maintain themselves. The hospital is small, but it has done, and is doing, admirable work; it was badly needed and has been most keenly appreciated. More than five hundred babies have been born there; there has been only one maternal death, and the infant mortality has been less than five per cent. The hospital has done much to suc-cour the poor population of Rheims. As an administrator of the civil hospitals of that city wrote:

You have been real 'Friends,' you have opened your doors wide to our orphans, our sick, our little children, whom you have come in person to fetch from the Martyr-City. Scorning danger, you have hastened in the thick of violent bombardment to take mothers on the point of their delivery into the refuge of your 'Maternity,' lavished on them all your care. Receive our eternal gratitude.

And indeed in the April of last year, this work of rescue from bombarded Rheims was work of no small danger as well as arduous in an extreme degree. In that month the little hospital housed for differing periods 334 refugees from Rheims and its neighbourhood, of ages from two months to eighty years. The city was then being systematically bombarded; and for three weeks the strain of this heavy work of evacuation on emergency went on. In two days four cars covered a distance of twelve hundred miles.

Mothers and children have often been living for a long period in cellars; a kind of existence that impoverishes the blood and sometimes brings about an almost total disinclination for food, besides predisposing the body to disease. Rest, fresh air, and proper nourishment do wonders by degrees to these sad cave-dwellers.

For convalescents, the Friends established a hospital at Sermaize and a home at Bettancourt. The Sermaize hospital consists of wooden huts with balconies, accommodating twenty to twenty-five patients. It is chiefly used as a convalescent home for delicate children of the neighbourhood; but during 1916 the addition of a couple of wards has made it possible to admit a certain number of women patients. Attending to out-patients also is a very important part of the work of the Sermaize Hospital. At Bettancourt, a château has been lent by a French lady, which serves as a home for children who are suffering from the ill effects of overcrowding and malnutrition. The children stay for several months as a rule, sometimes longer, and forty or fifty are housed there at a time. Both here and at Sermaize the improvement in the health of the children, save in very few cases, has been remarkable.

Another convalescent home was established by the Friends at Samoens in Haute Savoie. During the winter of 1915-16 nearly a hundred thousand persons returned to France through Switzerland. These *rapatriés* were families from the occupied districts who had been detained in Germany. They passed through Annemasse, where the invasion of these homeless folk created a great need for 'rest houses.' The French committees who were working for the *rapatriés* urgently asked the Friends to help; and with the assistance of the *Comité de Secours National* they took the Hotel Bellevue and its annexe at Samoens, near Annemasse. The hotel faces south, it is 2200 feet above the sea in a sun-bathed valley among the snowy mountains. Just as the home was ready, however, the stream of *rapatriés* stopped; and it was at once decided to use it for delicate women and children, specially chosen from among the refugees crowded in Paris slums. They quickly recover their health in the magnificent air, sleeping out on the balconies, with good food and watchful nursing. There are classes in English and embroidery, and drill for the children. Early in December 1916 the streams of *rapatriés* began to flow in again from Switzerland, at the rate of a thousand a day. They were sent on to join their relatives; but some of the sick and most suffering were taken in at Samoëns to rest and recover. During the past year a second convalescent home has been opened at Entremont in Haute Savoie as an overflow from Samoëns; but this hotel is not heated, and closes in October.

Lastly must be mentioned the labours of the district nurse at Troyes, for which the Mayor has expressed his gratitude, and those of the medical superintendent and district visitors among the refugees in Paris, who point out the dangers of overcrowding and conduct a vigilant campaign against its evils and the ever-threatening tuberculosis.

The work of the Friends in France has been, and is being, greatly augmented and extended through the coming of the United States into the war. American members of the society have already joined them in considerable numbers, principally men who are helping in the building and agricultural work. Any one who has had even a glimpse of the overwhelming and unlimited opportunities for aiding the patient, suffering legions of victims of the war in France will wish them from his heart a strong continuance and increase of support in their activities. For they come as men to men, and as women to women; they bring pity, but also respect; and in rebuilding homes they never forget that the main thing is to rebuild human dignity in those to whom an inhuman enemy has left nothing.

We have seen that the *rapatriés* are cared for not only at the Friends' hospitals in Haute Savoie, but also since the autumn of 1917 in the large hospital at Étrembières, endowed by New Zealand and managed by the *Comité Britannique,* which was described in its place.

Here may also be mentioned the work of a Scottish lady, who, backed by a committee in Glasgow, has carried out relief work in Flanders with devoted courage and perseverance; she has rescued hundreds of children from bombarded villages, both French and Flemish, and a great many of those she has placed in Switzerland, to be there housed and educated. She has also done much for homeless French and Flemish refugees, and for her noble service has received the *Croix de Guerre*.

In March 1917 a spasm of peculiar disgust ran through the civilised world. The Germans, retreating under the pressure of the Allies, carried out a rapid retreat from Bapaume and Péronne; and they left in the country thus 'freed' the most characteristic marks of their occupation. To wholesale thieving and burning; to the dynamiting, cottage by cottage, of every village; to the pulling down even of the just-ruined walls; to defacements, as fatuous as filthy, of things unvalued save for old feeling and association's sake – children's toys and dolls, photographs of absent ones in humble households; to such bestial usage of a peaceful and prosperous country-side, we had grown by degrees accustomed. It was what we looked for. But our advancing soldiers met a sight, that wintry March, for which they were not prepared. It was the sight of the fruit-trees deliberately sawn through above the roots, and lying prone, or, where there was not time to finish, deeply gashed all round.

Schadenfreude, 'joy in another's misfortune,' is a word peculiar to the German language, though common in German conversation. This ingenious crime, to which the murdered fruit-trees witnessed, seemed to have in it the leering triumph of the German *Schadenfreude* at its most triumphant.

A fruit-tree is one of earth's most beautiful things, with its apparition of pure blossom in the spring, and its clusters of ripe-coloured fruit in the later season; it has given, perhaps, of its abundance to one generation in the past, and will give to others hereafter. To kill was in itself a pleasure; but to murder defenceless and cherished beauty; to blast at once the present and the future; to rob unborn children as well as the helpless living; this, well thought out and relished in all its distant consequences, was a malignancy voluptuous to the baulked and retreating invader. ' France was never to rise again.'

To the rest of the world, unschooled in the philosophy of the German War Book, the act seemed strangely hideous. Like some other doings of this race, it seemed a spurting up of some aboriginal cruelty out of times before man was human, carried out as with the cold ritual of savage religions, yet guided by the trained will to hurt of military science.

Everywhere in the world where men till the kindly earth and live by its produce, this massacre of the fruit-trees was felt as a deep injury. It gave a new spur to the desire to help the inhabitants of those regions, and the suffering land itself. But long before this, at the beginning of the war, that desire had been strong among the farmers in England, and had found expression in action. When the Germans marched into France in August 1914, the peasantry were all busy with the harvest. But the crops were to be destroyed, the barns burnt, the machinery smashed, the population ruined.

To help in relieving all this distress, and re-establishing the farmers on their holdings, was a wish widespread and earnest among the farmers of this country.

The Royal Agricultural Society had in 1870 collected considerable sums for providing the farmers of France with seed corn in districts laid waste by the Germans. And now once more in 1915, the Society interpreted the feeling of the farmers of England by establishing a fund and a committee. The Agricultural Relief of Allies Committee found an opportunity of work immediately after the battle of the Marne, when a broad belt of land was recovered by the French. First, it sent a large consignment of agricultural machines and implements to replace those destroyed by the Germans. Then in the early summer of 1915 a considerable number of live stock was sent out; and later, seed wheat, seed oats, barley, and potatoes were supplied and distributed on the committee's behalf by the French Government, in the Department of the Marne, and also, in 1916, in the Verdun region.

Similar help in kind has been offered by English farmers through the committee, as each advance of the Allies has recovered territory from the enemy. Live poultry and rabbits have been given, as well as further gifts of seed. And close on ten thousand young fruit-trees, specially chosen for suitability to the soil and climate of the ruined districts, have been sent out to repair some of that malicious injury.

The farmers of the British Dominions have shown a growing practical interest in the fund – Canada especially. Representatives of agriculture in Canada, Australia, South Africa, and New Zealand have visited themselves the devastated districts, and have started campaigns in their own country on behalf of the French farmers.

The Royal Horticultural Society has also taken up the problem of reconstruction in the devastated districts; and the committee which it appointed has raised a large fund for the purpose, part of which is in course of distribution in France, while part is being reserved for use after the war.

Nor has the *Comité Britannique* neglected this problem, among its many spheres of operation; it has sent consignments of fruit-trees, and gives its aid in the plans for restocking and replanting.

In all this work the British Army on the spot has taken a vigorous hand, with keenly appreciated results. The French Academy of Agriculture has testified to the 'magnificent efforts of officers and men in the region conquered by their valour,' and has recorded how deeply touched the agriculturists of France have been, as well by the gifts of British agriculturists and their fraternal sympathy, as by the restoring achievements and devoted labours of the British soldiers.

Finally, a word must be said on the scheme set on foot by the *Comité Britannique* for establishing a farm colony in France, where soldiers threatened with tuberculosis may be treated. We have seen how terrible a problem is this of the spread of that malignant disease, and how vital it is for the future that it should be stayed. The proposed Farm Colony is to accommodate some 500 patients, and in its installation the results of the most modern discoveries will be embodied. Towards this scheme the British Farmers' Red Cross Fund, whose gift of a convoy has been noted in its place, has made the generous grant of £75,000.

Towards helping the general work of reconstruction, the *Comité Britannique* has opened a fund, to be employed when the hour is ripe. Its inspectors and commissioners continually collect information, with this design in view, so that field and orchard may be in due time reclaimed and new foundations laid upon the wreckage of the war. The *Comité* has also special funds for helping the various agencies in France which are labouring to mend the human waste; to train the maimed and the blinded, and to find them productive work.

PART III

IMPRESSIONS

ON THE FRONT IN CHAMPAGNE

It was what they call at the front a quiet day: a lull between two battles. The sky was overcast and dull. It was bad weather for observation, and no enemy 'sausages' overlooked the battle-ground; otherwise there would have been shells dropping all about the track by which we came.

The seared earth, patched here and there with splintered little pine-woods, rose opposite into a chain of bare hills. Each summit has a name, familiar in the story of the war for the obstinate battles waged upon its slopes, and not yet ended. I remembered the names from newspaper reports, and while reading had pictured them in my mind, quite different, as usually happens, from the reality. Each of these grey hills has run with blood. Only a few weeks before, the ground I looked on was in possession of the enemy and had been wrested from him by storm.

The landscape was, so to say, extinct. It had lost all its native life. The ground seemed inert, like the body of a dead creature under the claws of a fierce beast that shakes it now and then. It had convulsions of movement, not its own. Flashes shot out of the blank desolation. Shocks of sound thudded at one's ears. Shells rushed over, and after what seemed a long while burst in the distance. At intervals the short bark of field-guns diversified the noise. Black puffs and white puffs hung in the air above that forlorn range. But it was a quite desultory bombardment on either side. There seemed a kind of giant boredom about it, as of lions roaring in captivity. Men, as men, appeared no longer to exist. A vast and horrible impersonality pervaded this world, to which Dante's imagination might well have delighted to condemn the fussy and the self-important. Each shot, doubtless, was intended to hit something; but to a spectator without any inner knowledge there was an air of insanity, of unmotived persistence, of pure waste, about the whole grey scene, with its intermittent violence of sound.

Here was the ultimate tide-mark, the breaking surf, of those oceanic forces and activities which are moving so many nations to their depths. Statesmen in parliaments and on platforms, exhorting, explaining, defying; financiers with their myriads of clerks, spinning vast webs of figures; huge factories multiplying themselves everywhere, humming with machines, swarming with busy-fingered men and women; furnaces melting torrents of metal; the invisible energies everywhere; secret fervours of sacrifice; the glow of pure ideals, sustaining the hearts in tired bodies; passionate ambitions and corroding jealousies; rivers of hatred and resentment; the drill-sergeant on a thousand parade-grounds, ranks of boys moving at his bellow; girls eagerly learning the trades of their brothers; armies training, millions of young men disciplining their bodies to perfection of suppleness and hardness; women nursing and comforting the wreckage night and day; the very land tilled with a passion of anxious industry – all those vast and various populations at wrestle with Time, under the exaction of a single purpose, all that indescribable expenditure of spirit and flesh, ended here.

The mocking disparity seemed to shriek of futility and unreason. And so superior souls, dwelling above the battle, may moralise the world's situation. But the greater portent, greater than this seeming nightmare of abandonment to murder and madness, is this. Here is a war, waged by men who hate war; and yet they are persisting to the end.

The warriors of old who fought because they delighted in fighting, would never have endured what these men endure. Their spirit would have deserted them long ago.

Suddenly I experienced a sort of humiliation at coming on this scene as a spectator. The faint beginning of an intuition flashed through me of what the days and nights actually are to the soldier in the trenches. Miserable to an animal, what can this existence be to men accustomed to intelligent productive activity? Mud, wet, cold, discomfort, sameness, utter fatigue, vivid moments of danger, hideous hurts, torturing pain; the unendingness, the captivity, the single horizon – shrinking flesh and sensitive mind could never endure such prolongation of suffering, such paralysis of monotony, were they not sustained by the Idea which, dimly or clearly, assures them that this sound and fury, this idiot's tale, signified something.

The glory of man was never so great as in this war from which 'glory' has been banished. His spirit towers out of all the insane havoc and confusion, it is strong above death and destruction. It looks before and after; it sees what it desires; and for the sake of what belongs to its peace it shrinks from no extremity of pain.

Beyond that seared range of hills was all the opposed power of Germany, invisible but felt like an oppression. The enemy, too, suffers and endures; and him too an Idea sustains. Deep in the German mind is still throned that image, magnified as a shape in mist, of the blond Northern Hero, the conqueror and, by conquest, the benefactor, of inferior, softer, or degenerate peoples; the predestined inheritor of the world and its glory. It is true that in the plain light of day the heroic shape of dreams appears, for all his Wagnerian gestures and speeches, a grotesquely different figure; a book-keeping marauder, a bagman turned executioner, a shabby casuist over the victims of his careful murders, wordily plaintive when his deeds recoil upon him, if also resolute, scientific, resourceful, and armed with an indomitable will. But the Idea has intoxicated a people by nature preferring their own conceptions to experience; and it is still stronger than themselves. Those who sit above the battle and those who would appeal to moral forces make a vast error, when they argue as if it were merely a case of primitive violence let loose. It is one moral force against another. Our reason is the enemy's unreason. What to us is the world's desire and hope is to them a contemptible dream. It is a creed we fight against – a creed acted out with a logical thoroughness and passion such as few religions in history have inspired.

A cheerful voice was saying at my ear: 'I suppose we had better not pass in front of this battery, as it is just going to fire.'

A warning arm shot up from the gun-pits. The car swerved abruptly from the rough track, and turned at right angles over a narrow bridge of poles and turf which spanned the trench.

We were now safely behind the battery; and as we passed, the 75's, under their roof of boughs, began to fire. One had a glimpse of their recoil and lunge, a movement which had something animal-like in its lithe swiftness. That famous weapon, which has no imposing size, but which is such a marvel of precision and rapidity, has become a symbol for the French, just as it seems to typify their qualities. More than one soldier has said to me that the Marne was the victory of the *Soixante-Quinze*; and the enthusiasm for the personality of the gun (so to speak) is universal in the population. I could understand it.

A little farther on we crossed the trench again by another narrow bridge, just wide enough for the car.

'Not too easy to find on a dark night without lamps!'

'But how do you do it at all?'

'Oh, one gets an instinct.'

I could only marvel. But my companion, the second in command of Section 1 of the S.S.A., one of the British Ambulance Committee's Convoys, nonchalantly guided his car over the roughest ground, and had evidently long ceased to wonder at his own skill.

We got out of the car at a ragged pine-wood, to visit one of the advanced posts. The ground was strewn with old cartridge-cases, rusty iron, and other suchlike débris of the recent battle; accentuating somehow the desolateness of the landscape and the day.

One of the section was at the post, with his car waiting. He greeted us with a gesture of disappointment: 'Nothing doing!'

The gunners alone seemed busy, and the ambulances had no work for the moment.

At the other post we had some talk with the French soldiers. One of them, a sergeant, went out with us a little way, and pointed out the opposite crests by name, and the salient features of the ground, and what had been the old German lines over which the French had advanced a month before. And listening to this sergeant with his face of fine intelligence, and his lucid exposition, one began to remember, under all the horror and unnatural boredom, the intellectual vigilance that a vast organised effort demands for its comprehension; the subtle co-ordination of detail, where to the mere spectator everything seems an intricate confusion; above all, one caught something of that fusing glow of faith in France, that most human yet almost divine determination to go on to the end in a cause that possesses body and spirit alike.

This sergeant was an *abbé*.

At the *Poste de Secours* they showed us with great pride a just-completed system of pipes from which hot water could be had in a few minutes. We passed through the dressing station, with its double exit, contrived in case of blocking by a shell. One or two soldiers with fresh slight wounds were waiting, or being bandaged. We stumbled and slipped about the trenches on the chalky slime : and I could faintly imagine, if this was the effect of one day's rain, of what abominable mire the Champagne soil was capable after weeks of continuous downpour. Up those slippery slopes, in full exposure to the enemy fire, the French had swept forward in wild showers of sleet last month. It was on roads of such slime, broken into great pits, that our English convoys worked day and night, without lamps, among the crowded and interminable traffic of the transport, during both the great battles of Champagne.

A CANTEEN IN THE FOREST

For a moment one might have thought it a mist of blue-bells among the beeches.

Gliding down the road in a sunny silence through the green forest, the car turned to the right up an incline, and we found ourselves among the trucks and grassy sidings of a little railway station. Then the patches of misty blue among the trees – for the whole place was a clearing in great woods – explained themselves. It was the uniform of *Poilus*, lying at ease in the shade. Passing some sheds, we were met by the sight of a great crowd of blue-uniformed soldiers, many hundreds of them sitting, standing, or lying down, and grouped thickest about the shed opposite to which the car drew up.

There was a great opening in the side of the shed, and there, pouring out coffee for the men gathered in front, and chatting pleasantly with them, was an Englishwoman, the *Directrice* of the canteen. As it happened, it was a lady whom I knew. The last time I had talked with her was on the stage of a London theatre. Now, in white uniform, she was dispensing coffee and lemonade and cigarettes to the French soldiers, as she had been doing for many months past, at more than one canteen. With a warm greeting, she called her husband (he happens to be a famous actor), who was filling great jugs of coffee from big boilers inside the shed, and with a hail of surprise he emerged and shook hands.

It was the first of our canteens that I had seen. The delegate of the *Comité Britannique*, who supervises the organisation of the *Cantines des Dames Anglaises* at the headquarters in the Boulevard Magenta, and makes smooth the relations between the English workers and the French authorities, had driven me out to Orry-la-Ville (the village which gives its name to the railway station) in his car. And while he discussed details and supplies, I took in the scene around me.

A continuous stream of soldiers passed in front of the canteen, and the lady serving them had not a moment's rest from her talk. She poured out coffee and lemonade without ceasing, and at the same time chatted with the men as they came up. They smiled their greetings, often adding a compliment or a joke; and sometimes a group lingered while they drank their coffee, and talked about the war or about themselves.

I imagined to myself the labour of perpetually pouring out cups of coffee for hours together, and felt sympathetic aches in the muscles of my arm. This is no light work that these English ladies are doing; and if you remember that, whatever the fatigue, it is a point of honour to be always interested, cheerful, smiling, you will admire them as whole-heartedly as I do.

'How many men do you serve with refreshments, as a rule?' I asked.

'About twelve hundred an hour.'

I looked round in the sunshine, and essayed a rough con-jecture of the numbers of the soldiers gathered about in the clearing; but I soon gave it up, too much interested in the men themselves.

The most of my acquaintance with the Poilu had been in hospital. When I thought of him, there came before me the picture of a figure in pyjamas and slippers, or with oddments of uniform : gentle-mannered, sometimes rather grim-looking, but oftener bright-eyed, and quick with a charming smile, even in the midst of pain; with nothing about him to suggest drills and parade-grounds; a very human person, with a good deal of the child in his nature.

Here were the same types, but healthy, active: fairhaired men from Picardy, blue-eyed swarthy Bretons; long, silent Normans; quick-witted, voluble '*Parigots*'; here and there an Arab; olive-complexioned men from the Midi; smooth-cheeked lads and ruddy, bearded Territorials; all in blue, except for the occasional mustard khaki of the Colonial troops, with their dull blue helmets on their heads – lighter and better shaped than the English 'tin hat,' though possibly less protective – all burnt with the sun, and gathered in knots that dissolved into strolling movement and collected again, as they passed to and from the canteen or stretched themselves on the ground, or stood and talked, or sat and smoked in silence.

The fresh green of the beeches lit up by contrast the moving blue of the uniforms and the brown glow of the faces.

I wanted to question the *Directrice* about her experiences, but would not interrupt that beneficent labour of libation, and could only exchange a word or two with her on her work. She was enthusiastic about the soldiers. She had got to know many of them well; they had told her their histories, and what poignant tales these were!

It is only by talking with the French soldiers that an Englishman can realise what the war is to France – especially what it means to be invaded. Not only to wake every morning with the consciousness that the enemy is there, in your own country – a consciousness of insult and pollution – but it may be to have had no news of your wife, your parents, and children, only to know that they are in the power of the Germans.

What wonder that sometimes a passing cloud of depression descends on these soldiers, who have been fighting so long? It is in the times of waiting that they are most liable to such fits; and therefore the work of the canteens is of inestimable value. It is not only refreshments, it is still more the friendly talk, the games, impromptu entertainments, and tunes such as the soldiers delight in from the handy gramophone. Their spirits easily react. I was told of a wonderful singer, a Poilu himself, I believe, who had sung his comrades into heart again with his songs, and had spoken also and fired them with his own passionate faith. But just now they were in great distress at the canteen. The gramophone had broken down. Was it possible to get it mended in Paris, or to hire a new one?

While the wounds of the gramophone were being discussed, I turned to the soldiers. One had a dog with him, a small terrier of some sort. I asked if he was taking it to the trenches. 'Oh yes, that's his home. He has done his two years in the trenches.'

'Quite a veteran. How old is he?'

'Ah, who knows? We found him in the trench, when we occupied it first. We kill the Boches, and he kills the rats.'

'And where are you fighting now?'

'St-Quentin. Next to the English.'

The other men had come up, and we were naturally curious to hear what the French soldier thought of his English comrade.

A tall, straight-standing corporal, bronzed, with grave, level eyes, gave us some details of what was actually going on about St-Quentin; and he spoke of the English soldiers.

He praised them quietly, but heartily, with professional appreciation. We praised the French in our turn, and the unique qualities which have made their armies famous.

'But you are more dogged than we are – you took Vimy Ridge.'

'Yes, we took Vimy Ridge, it is true, but after all'

'We failed.'

One could not deny that Vimy had been stormed by the Canadians and British; but we wanted to express our conviction that no soldiers in the world surpass the French. And, at any rate, we could dwell on all that our new armies had learnt from the armies of France.

Certainly, since the Somme battles began, there is a new feeling about the English in France. For a long time there was a certain bewilderment. There was so much talk of Britain's millions of soldiers, and so little appeared to be attempted by them. It was hard, in a country habituated to military service, to understand that these new armies needed time to get ready for actual fighting. But now it is different, and appreciation of our soldiers is generously given.

The *Directrice* at Orry has presided over canteens in more than one part of France, and she and her husband have had rich opportunities for making friends with the *Poilus*, for one of the canteens was at a *Dépôt des Éclopés* or Rest Dépôt, where the soldiers are not, as at the railway stations, birds of brief passage, but stay for a number of days. They told me of the *Poilus'* first impressions of the Tommy. So false can legendary tradition be that he was expected to be gloomy and self-absorbed. But then that marvel of cheerfulness, resource, and good nature appeared and dissolved this shadowy myth in his own warm reality. 'Why, they would share their last biscuit with us!' But how rash were the English! What impossible things they would do! And how *chic* their dying – with a laugh on their lips!'

It was time to be going. There was a crowd now near the canteen, where the *Directrice* still poured coffee with the smiling patience of a Naiad in an old print pouring from her never-exhausted urn. Shouts and laughter came from the crowd, and as they parted for a moment one could see that they were absorbed in a game. Merely throwing little rings on to pegs in a small board hung on the shed; but what matters the apparatus or the object? A game is a game; and there is no medicine like a game for tired and fretted minds, for thoughts that drive in grooves of memory and pain.

I had noticed a little earlier a soldier who had diverted his thoughts in another way, and, though a magistrate might not have decided him to be drunk, he was overflowing in his gestures and expressions. Such things, I was told, were very infrequent. But what struck me was not this, but the action of his comrade, who was endeavouring to calm him by appealing to his courtesy. He was not to show himself thus before the English lady who had come to wait upon their wants. And his appeal succeeded.

HOSPITALS IN AND ABOUT PARIS

We had come that morning from Royaumont. People, I suppose, used to visit Royaumont in peace time, as they go to see Tintern in England, and Jumièges in Normandy, and Villers-la-Ville in Belgium, and beautiful ruins of old abbeys anywhere. But now they visit Royaumont not because it is a ruined abbey, but because it is the one hospital for the wounded in France entirely managed and staffed by women. On an earlier page I have described this great enterprise of the Scottish women, and have said something of the difficulties they so gallantly defeated in taking over and adapting to use the old buildings which St-Louis saw rise in their first grandeur – the Abbey was founded by his mother, Blanche of Castille – and the stones of which he had helped to lay in their places with his own hands.

The Abbey Church is now a ruin, or hardly even that, so little is left of it. The great pillars of the nave are sawn away close to the turf which now floors the aisles, all open to the sky. But the cloisters, and the rest of the vast monastic buildings, restored in parts, remain. And there are streams and fishponds and fruit-trees. There is a sense of old and large abundance in the surroundings, the heritage of peaceful centuries. One has distant green glimpses of the forests beyond.

On this May morning, when the cherry was in clouds of white bloom, the impression was one of singular peace and beauty. And at once on entering the abbey one receives a sensation of airy cleanness and of order. To know what condition the buildings had been in three years ago, and to see them now, was to marvel at the wonders that energetic feminine hands had wrought.

On an upper floor we were received by the distinguished woman-surgeon who is the *Médecin-chef*, and taken over the hospital. All is spacious and on a stately scale. The old refectory, where St-Louis used to minister to the monks and taste their wine, is now a ward that holds a hundred beds. All the wards are roomy and pleasant. But what lingers most vividly in the memory is the cloisters. They enclose a rose-garden, in the centre of which is a fountain. And roofing the cloisters is a broad terrace, running round the square of them and overlooking the garden. Beds can be moved out of the wards on to this terrace; and numbers of the wounded were there, lying or sitting in the sun; others basked in the garden below.

Convalescents strolled about the grounds. A boat had been provided for them, and a merry party were pushing off into the stream. Some were angling in the lake. Few Frenchmen are not enthusiastic fishermen; and to be allowed to practise their gentle sport is a precious solace in the long weariness of getting well. Infinite tedium succeeding to cruel suffering! And yet these French soldiers, with their fine elasticity of mind and body, their capacity of being interested and amused by small things of the passing hour, bear it all with quiet fortitude, and have a ready smile.

At Royaumont I was struck with the order and discipline that prevailed. The very fact that there are no men in authority over them appeals to the chivalry of the French nature. It is all the more a point of honour to impose a duty on themselves. One had a sense of happy co-operation between the patients and the staff.

And for the staff, and the work they have done, what can one say sufficient? The women of Scotland have cause to be proud of these their representatives, who surely will leave a fragrant memory behind them in Royaumont. For it is not only the wounded, but the inhabitants of the hamlets round about, deprived of medical aid by the war's necessities, to whom they minister. The sick and hurt of the neighbourhood, under sanction of the French authorities, get care and comfort from the Scottish nurses.

The staff is large, and needs to be so, in so vast a place. Besides the doctors and sisters and nurses, there are those who look after the clothing of the soldiers. A big job, this! The clothes of the new arrivals must be sorted, the linen washed, everything numbered and entered in a card-index; and then there is the mending. As in most of these hospitals, French workers from the neighbourhood help. At Royaumont they undertake the mending of the linen; but the mending of the uniforms is done by the Scottish women, who take a special pride in the cleanness and good repair of the soldiers' equipment when it is handed back to them on their evacuation. They bear testimony to the French soldier's cleanliness and to the wonderful excellence of his linen. 'What needlewomen the French wives and sisters must be!' writes one of the ladies in charge of the *Vêtement*. This lady, in the early days, used to carry up the sacks of clothing to the fifth-storey attics on her back. But another member of the staff devised a block-pulley, by which they are now hauled up – an immense lightening of labour. Other instances of inventive resource met us as we went over the hospital. In an upper room, devoted to massage and the exercising of stiffened limbs – *mécanothérapie* as the doctors call it – I noticed a dwarf harmonium and a sewing-machine. I asked what they were for; and was told that they had been found in the abbey building and impressed into the hospital service. For exercising arms and feet both these instruments were discovered to be as admirable as the most costly and up-to-date apparatus.

But everywhere the eye for details, the care for comely neatness, were apparent.

If any male doubt the capacity of women to organise, administrate, and create a cheerful order, let him go to Royaumont.

But Royaumont, as has been told already, is not the only witness to the ancient tie of friendship between France and Scotland.

I went one afternoon in Paris to seek out the *Hôpital de l'Écosse*. The Rue de la Chaise is a retired street, a little off the Boulevard Raspail on the left bank of the Seine; and there, in an old mansion with a courtyard and high gateway on the street – which before the war was the nursing-home of a well-known Paris doctor, now the hospital's director – I found the hospital. The Doctor, for whom I asked, was out, but was expected shortly. I was invited to wait in the garden, and, passing through the spacious courtyard, was led through the building to the back. Here, to my surprise, was a large garden, like the fragment of a park; and so sequestered was it by the high walls on either side and the great old trees within it, that, as I sat and watched the white clouds over the leafy chestnuts, Paris, which was around me, with its noise and traffic, seemed remote and unreal.

Wounded officers and soldiers were lying or sitting on the terrace in front of the tall windows of the ground floor ward or under the trees, and strolled or limped among the shrubberies beyond the lawn. Nurses came with smiling looks, and talked to them as they passed in or out. Some had little knots of friends or relatives about them. A singular peacefulness was in the air.

A hospital in the midst of a great city is not what one would choose to come to, if one were wounded; yet here, with the scents of early summer all about, and so much delightful foliage, it seemed as if it would be hard to find a more reposeful haven.

It was a pleasant place to sit and muse in. But it is ill thinking in war time, and in a hospital. One must be doing, or the thought of all the maimed youth and the dead rises to choke one with pity and anger at the unpardonable madness of it all.

The director had been delayed. I waited till I could wait no longer. And then, at last, just as I was leaving, he arrived and met me in the gateway. I had chosen the afternoon as the best time for visiting, when the surgeons are more at leisure. But the Doctor would not hear of my seeing over the hospital at such a time. No, it must be seen *en pleine activité* – that is, in the morning; and a morning was to be fixed for my visit.

So, a week or two later – for several long though hurried journeys were to intervene – I again presented myself at the Rue de la Chaise, and the Doctor, with genial pride, introduced me to the full activity of the hospital.

Almost the first thing I remarked was the wonderful absence of those familiar medical odours which one associates with hospital wards. The Doctor was gratified; it was a point on which he felicitated himself and his staff. And next I was struck by the stateliness and beautiful proportions of the rooms. The house is in the grand style of the old regime. It belonged at one time to Pauline Bonaparte

– the beautiful sister of Napoleon; and portraits of that period still hang on the tall panels in one of the rooms, over the beds of the wounded. The largest ward is in what was the old chapel of the building, a great, vaulted place with long rows of beds on either side, endowed by gifts from Scotland. Running along the garden terrace, with French windows opening on it, is a group of sunny wards, opening into each other. The outlook on the garden, and the sunshine, made these particularly pleasant; and the patients evidently found them so. The nurses I met were some of them French, others Scottish and Irish; the doctors and surgeons are French – men with famous names and distinguished masters in their profession. All the equipment seemed of the most modern and complete. We found many of the wounded busily occupied in making little baskets and ornaments and toys. Some of them had become highly skilful in this dainty manufacture; and when I left, the director pressed on my acceptance some charming specimens of their work. And in a glass of the delicious wine of Anjou, the Doctor's own country, we drank to the mutual affection and friendship of France and Britain. Indeed, this hospital has been a centre for the expansion of the Cordial Understanding. The Doctor has neglected no opportunity to secure speakers and lecturers to celebrate fitting occasions by interpreting the ideals and the efforts of the two nations to each other. Actors and actresses from the Comédie Française have recited versions of English poems; and the band of the English Guards has played in the courtyard for the pleasure of the wounded.

Before leaving, I was shown a sort of annexe to the hospital, where Belgian soldiers passing through Paris can obtain a rest and a meal.

On another morning I was taken out of Paris to the hospital at Ris-Orangis. We left Paris by the Porte de Versailles, and drove along the straight stone-paved roads, where the tall poplars had in a day or two sprung into such exquisitely tinted leaves. We admired the golden flush of the foliage, while we execrated the pave.

Ris-Orangis lies south-west of Paris, at a distance of about twenty kilometres.

As we approached the village, the blossom of orchards and the rising woods behind made an attractive prospect. And when we had arrived at the College, which a thorough renovation has turned into so fine a hospital, we found the surroundings even pleasanter than they promised. The park, with its woods and banks, its slopes of sward and winding walks, has a richness of varied views and abundance of sunny and sheltered places, admirable for convalescence. And the hospital itself has been fitted out with magnificent completeness. The X-Ray apparatus is one of the finest in France. The hospital is famous, too, for the suspensory treatment of fractures which has been practised there with so much success. The building, with its wide and airy corridors – and narrow passages, such as are often found in improvised hospitals, are no joy to stretcher-bearers – has proved well adapted to its purpose; but both it and the park had fallen into neglect, and were only brought into this present spotless order by much labour and at great expense. We lunched with the staff. There was only one lament – that they were not receiving as many wounded as they wanted. And, indeed, it seemed a pity that these beautiful spacious wards should not be always occupied as long as there were wounded coming from the front, and that such lavish equipment and such resources of skill and care should not be utilised to the full.

The garage is a very important part of the establishment at Ris-Orangis, as the cars work for a whole circuit of hospitals in the neighbourhood. We visited the garage and inspected the cars before leaving. On the way I saw some brown tents of an unusual pattern in the grounds. They were, I was told, American Army tents, which are used for patients needing open-air treatment; and they were said to have served this purpose signally well.

RUINS AND REFUGEES

I do not know which impresses the mind more in travelling about Eastern France – the violence and thoroughness of the destruction in the ruined villages, or the way in which the land has been kept under cultivation. In places where there seems to be no population left, you will find the vast fields tilled and the crops growing. It is true the tillage is nothing like what it was in times of peace; a practised eye will mark the pathetic difference; crops are invaded by all sorts of insolent weeds; but the effort is there, the undefeated effort. Sometimes you may see an old man, bent but active, or a couple of old women, burnt by the sun, labouring slowly and without pause in an else solitary landscape, of which they seem to have become a part. Truly there is a homely heroism in this stubborn persistence of the French peasant – though the shells are falling in his field, he keeps his plough to the furrow – which is strangely moving. The kindly earth has never failed him or his fathers, and it will not fail him now. He is a figure of mute faith, stronger than the violence of kings or than the cannonade of armies.

Precisely a hundred years before the war began, in the early days of August 1814, an English traveller wrote from Troyes in Champagne:

> We came 120 miles in four days; the last two days we passed over the country that was the seat of war. I cannot describe to you the frightful desolation of the scene; village after village entirely ruined and burned, the white ruins towering in innumerable

293

forms of destruction among the beautiful trees. The inhabitants were famished; families once independent now beg their bread in this wretched country; no provisions, no accommodation, filth, misery, and famine everywhere.

The English traveller was Shelley; the description occurs in that amazing letter to the wife whom he had just deserted, in which he invites her to join him and Mary Godwin in Switzerland. Harriet, we may guess, was far from being interested in such descriptions. But for any one who travels through the desolated regions of France to-day, that passage comes with a curiously vivid reality. A hundred years, and the land which had long recovered its old bounteous tranquillity, as if nothing had ever shaken it, is again defaced and spoiled; and this time with far mightier engines of ruin, and with a yet more pitiless extortion from its inhabitants. Only those who have seen it can realise a tithe of what it means – and of what we in England have been spared. The Germans also!

In a little bare upper room of an ancient house in Troyes I visited a grey-haired couple, refugees from a village in the region beyond Châlons. The old woman was blind. She sat in her chair, felt for my hand, and took it and kissed it, 'because I was English.' 'Ah, yes!' said the old man, 'it is true; the English have saved our lives.' And he told me, and his wife corroborated him with a word and a nod from time to time, how they were overtaken by the war and driven homeless along the roads till at last they came to be housed and cared for by the Society of Friends. They lived in a valley, in a quiet village. They knew what war was, for they had lived through 1870. But for all that, though they knew that the Germans were again invading their country, and were very near, the villagers remained in their homes; they refused to believe that any harm would come to them. ' But this is no war,' said the old man. It was something one could not have believed in. Suddenly, in the sunshine, crash out of nowhere came a shell, and the church steeple toppled into ruin. The terrified inhabitants took to their cellars. ' I told them they would not be harmed,' said the old man. ' But I did not know what kind of a war this was.'

They heard in their cellars the smashing of roofs and windows; then came the tramp of soldiers and shouted orders; the enemy was in the street. The villagers were summoned up; and then – if a man did not salute, if he failed to answer at once, if he did not say just what they wanted him to say, at a nod from an officer he was put against the wall and shot in a trice. 'No, no, this is no war, not as men used to make war.'

Yet this was a village where the Germans had been by comparison mild. Multiply the villages by hundreds; call up the country-side in England round your home, or the country you know and love best; number over the hamlets and farms with their familiar names and kind associations; picture them all blackened and broken in pieces, and the old people in the cottages driven out in miserable troops along strange roads to beggary among strangers, shot dead on any provocation or dying in ditches from hunger and weakness; and you will begin to understand. But only begin. For the extent of the desolation passes the power of description. The mind would become blunted by the monotony of havoc, horror, and misery, before a fraction of the tale were told. If a human heart were capable of comprehending a thousandth part of the suffering and waste of the war in its reality – that is, as it comprehends its own griefs – it would burst with pity, shame, and indignation.

The Germans have carried out with a simple faith the precepts of their War Book, the precepts reiterated by all their venerated teachers of the science of war. Civilian inhabitants must be intimidated and made to suffer by every possible means and with no least atom of weak mercy.

Thus they will create a moral atmosphere in the invaded nation which will cause it speedily to sue for peace.

The logic seems faultless; it has been dutifully acted out, with the most scrupulous correctness and precision – very often against all natural inclination – with a thoroughness which is *echt deutsch*; yet the conclusion does not come as it should. Nothing enrages the German mind like a syllogism gone wrong. The syllogism must be right, because it is the product of German thought; something eke must bear the blame. And in the full-blown savagery of destruction to which certain places in France bear immortal witness, the rage of exasperated intellect in the command has combined with bestial instinct in the soldiery to do things no one would have believed that men would do to men. But the greatness of man lives in a world beyond logic. It endures beyond calculation, and prevails over all that the cruelty of reason can contrive.

It was in the pleasant valley of the Mortagne, a little river that runs northwards to the Meuse, as we drove towards Nancy, that we came into the region of the devastations. A barn at the corner of the road, tumbled into a shapeless heap; then a hamlet, shattered and deserted, with pitiful remnants of its old quiet felicity; gaping walls burnt purple, loop-holed and bespattered with bullet-marks; such sights were soon so frequent that the eyes passed over them, only noting when the relic of a family, still clinging to the last of home, stared up from a doorstep, and a dog barked in the solitude of the street. But all around was the green, sweet country; and everywhere, this miraculous May, the abounding blossom was radiant on the fruit-trees.

The black ruins and the white blossom haunted one's mind; my thoughts were full of the young who were dead, fallen in their faith and cause, and lying now in how many thousands of graves under the earth of their own country, that spread before me in the spring sunshine. It seemed to my fancy that they had risen again in that triumphant blossom, to reassure the world.

We were entering the district over which were fought momentous battles in August and September 1914. The German armies, making their great effort to break through the French line between Toul and Epinal, were here held and stopped. Had the invaders succeeded, they might well have achieved their aim of enveloping the main French forces from the south, as it was the aim of other German armies to envelop them on the north; hence the vital import of the struggle. To and fro, from town to town, and village to village, the obstinate conflict was fought, till at the decisive moment the enemy was driven back.

It is the bitter necessity of the defenders of an invaded country to join with the enemy in maiming what is their own. The difference is that the one side does all it can to spare, the other does all it can to destroy. French shells, as well as German, have played some part in making these poor ruins. But the most significant desolation of this region is by no means the work of mere fighting.

My companion said to me: 'We are approaching Gerbéviller.' The name struck on my mind with a sense of shadowy horror. I remembered the story of Gerbéviller.

Soon we were in the main street of what was once so pleasant a small town, set upon the banks of three branching streams, and passed slowly between the rows of ruins. The place was bombarded by the Germans, and afterwards by the French; but what we saw was no random wreckage, it was the relics of a scientific and complete destruction. Here was the bridge over the Mortagne, flowing in the clear sunshine beside this strange dead human silence, the bridge on which the remnant of the little body of defenders – sixty or seventy strong – held out behind a barricade against the overwhelming odds of Bavarians. As far as can be ascertained, most of these got away during the night, but a few, separated from the rest, could only escape by killing a German sentry in their way. The sentry's body was found in the morning by the German's; they insisted that he had been killed by the inhabitants, and for a punishment set fire to the whole place, house by house, with the pastilles carried with them for such purposes, and 'executed' a number of the old and helpless inhabitants with hideous indignities. The remnant of the population was entirely homeless, when the French drove the retreating Germans out of the town. The Préfet of the Department of Meurthe-et-Moselle visited Gerbéviller while the ruins were still smoking, and blackened skeletons still lay among the charred ruins; and on his second visit he took with him an English correspondent, Mr. Gerald Campbell, who has given an account of what happened, and of what he saw himself, in his book *Verdun to the Vosges*. But the story of Gerbéviller-La-Martyre is known to every Frenchman, not only for the savage things done there, but still more for the shining courage and devotion of the famous Sister Julie and the little band of Sisters of Mercy who worked with her during those August days of horror.

Gerbéviller has the pre-eminence of desolation, but it is only one place among how many!

And now think for a moment what all these wrecked towns and obliterated villages mean. What armies of the beggared and the homeless! France has on her hands over two million refugees from the devastated districts. How and where are they to be housed, fed, clothed, comforted, employed?

Two years before, in the summer of 1915, at Sermaize-les-Bains, in the Department of the Marne, which is a scene of ruin wellnigh as complete as Gerbéviller itself, I had a glimpse of the work that is being done in the devastated districts by the Society of Friends, side by side with various French organisations, and with the help and sanction of the Government.

It was just a year after the battles of the Marne. Among the forlorn remains of the destroyed town new clusters of neat wooden huts and brick cottages were springing up. It was like a colony of settlers building on some ancient ruins; for these destroyed towns and villages might be of any age; they belong to Death, who keeps no dates. A group of Quaker workers stood in a line tossing bricks from one to another with the deft rapidity of practised bricklayers, where a cottage was nearing completion. A woman invited me into her cottage, and showed it to me with a certain pride and pleasure, in spite of the calamities into which the war had thrown her. I talked with some of the Friends in their own hut, and found them very eager upon their work, especially upon the human side of it. They felt their real reward was when they had succeeded in implanting some seed of hope and care for the future in the stunned hearts of those homeless ones.

For the frightful suddenness of the blow had been a paralysing shock. There was no warning, no preparation. The first shell burst close to the church on Sunday during Mass, just at the moment of the elevation of the Host; yet the cure finished the Mass. After the wave of war had passed, leaving the town in ruins, there were numbers of the inhabitants, here as elsewhere, who crept back to the place; and families were found living in what were cellars, with a makeshift roof to shelter them, the smoke from the stove they had contrived to introduce going up in the midst of the chaos of desolation, to witness to that passionate clinging to home which the French have so strongly. If these forlorn and stricken people could have had all the world to choose from, they would still have chosen the spot that, wrecked, burnt-out, and defaced, alone meant home for them. For these unhappy families the huts and cottages of the Friends, and still more their encouraging presence and sympathy, were indeed comfort and support.

At Gerbéviller, a few months after its destruction, the Friends helped the Préfet of Meurthe-et-Moselle, at his request, by making an inventory of all goods belonging to the refugees. They had already done the same service at Reméréville, and had administered relief in a number of villages of the Department. But this work had all been completed early in 1916.

As has been told already, there are numbers of refugees collected in the city of Troyes, the old capital of Champagne. They have streamed down southwards and westwards from the Ardennes; pitiable and bewildered processions, pushing hand-carts with their hastily snatched belongings piled upon them, or carrying in their hands whatever a wild instinct had prompted them to save – objects sometimes of a pathetic and absurd unlikeliness. One sad lady found herself, to her own subsequent bewilderment and dismay, clasping three umbrellas, the sole treasure rescued from her household goods.

I came to Troyes one morning and sought out the headquarters of the Friends; and the officer in charge was my hospitable guide in a little journey of exploration through the town.

Troyes is a city of fine Gothic architecture; of picturesque corners; of narrow alleys, where the gabled houses lean toward each other across the way in their extreme old age; a place to rejoice the heart of an etcher, and to make a sanitary surveyor stand aghast. Every here and there one finds a little stream, an outlet from the Seine, which winds through the town, gliding along the back walls of old stooping houses; and one sees women kneeling to wash clothes in the running water. To find decent accommodation for refugees in an old town like this, the population of which had been so much swollen since the war began, was no easy matter. Owing to the crowded conditions and the great demand for rooms, rents were exorbitantly high. The Society of Friends had constructed a large number of movable wooden huts, built to a pattern, in an open space on the outskirts, when, owing to the Allies' advance in the spring of 1917 and the liberation of a great tract of country, these huts had to be given up to the more pressing necessity of providing shelters for refugees in the Noyon district. What was to be done? It happened that there were a certain number of old houses marked for demolition. As these were better than nothing for the time being, the Friends arranged with the civil authorities for the postponement of their demolition, and housed several families in each. Besides this, the representatives of the Society supply cheap furniture – chairs and simple wardrobes – made on the spot; and this they sell at a very low price on the instalment system. Also bedding and clothes. I saw piles, of mattresses in store-rooms, and feather-beds in process of being filled; and in another part of the town saw a shop full of chairs and wardrobes, neat pieces of plain carpentry, unpainted.

As we walked through those ancient streets, passing the church where our Henry the Fifth wedded his French Kate, I noted how often my companion was greeted with smiles and shining eyes, and we stopped to exchange a word with one or other of the refugees; I remember especially a mother with her child whom she had lost for two whole years (the father had been shot), and who was now restored to her.

We visited some of the families lodged in the houses that had been procured for them. It was in one of these that we found that old couple whose story I have already told. Others were young, though they had memories enough to fill a lifetime. I heard their histories; full of terrors and hairbreadth escapes, and violent partings and strange unhoped-for meetings. g But here in their quiet rooms, with the sunlight falling on the floor, they were busy with their occupations – dressmaking, tailoring, or what not. For it is the aim of the Friends to find work for the refugees – by preference of course the work to which they have been bred. What so blessed as the dulling solace of regular daily work for those who have so vivid a nightmare behind them?

Yet, for all that has been done and is doing, how immense and dark is this world of dislocated existences! Its immensity haunts the mind, it makes the heart sore.

LYONS AND NEVERS

It was six o'clock of a cloudless morning when I alighted at Lyons from the Paris express.

Breakfast over, I asked for the Ulster Hospital. I was told it was a long way off, and advised to take a carriage. Carriages, however, seemed extremely scarce. The immense tree-planted square in front of the Perrache station was still full of the booths of the great Lyons Fair, which had recently been held. Here I sought for a fly, but none was visible; and it was a long time before one appeared and consented to take me to my destination. Crossing the Rhone, I was driven down many long streets and leafy boulevards to the outlying suburb, where at last we turned in to the Allée du Sacré Cœur, and I saw the legend Ulster Volunteer Hospital, No. 250 bis.

The building which has been taken over for the hospital was a technical school. It has large and pleasant rooms which serve for wards, but otherwise is not fitted with much in the way of modern comfort and convenience. All shortcomings, however, of this kind had been overcome by the energy of the staff. There was evidence of inventive improvisation; and every opportunity was turned to account. The *Médecin-chef* gave me a cordial welcome, and we went the round of the wards. It was easy to see that the happiest relations prevailed between staff and patients. The Poilu was among friends. An Irish gaiety and animation were in the air. A great cherry-tree thick with exquisite white blossom, just outside the window of one of the wards, seemed to be flowering expressly for the pleasure of the wounded. I talked with some of these, and found them all more than contented with their quarters and the care bestowed on them. The hospital contains a hundred beds. It was three-quarters full, and more wounded were expected.

The *Directrice* invited me to lunch, in company with some of the nurses, at a modest, tiny, but amusing and excellent restaurant a few doors off, to which the staff are in the habit of adjourning. Afterwards we were to drive across the city to the other British hospital at St-Rambert.

I was told about the move from Pau, where the Ulster Hospital was originally set up, and heard experiences of those early days of the war.

A motor ambulance came round from the garage to take me across the town. It was an opportunity for a joy-ride for some of the more convalescent soldiers; and with a good deal of merriment and raillery among themselves, and friendly comments and commands from the nurses, they were collected for the outing and helped each other in. The *Directrice* (whose French is of an enviable perfection) gave her orders, punctiliously obeyed by the soldiers, and took her seat at the wheel. We called at a suburban station to see if there were any wounded expected by the train for the hospital, but none were arriving that day. It is usually arranged for the tram, which passes close to the hospital, to bring the sitting cases.

Our way led us across both the Rhone and the Saône, the two noble streams which curve through the city and unite below it. At the other extremity of the town and beyond its suburbs is the island of St-Barbe, a resort of holiday-makers lying in the stream of the Saône; and a little nearer the city, on a steep and wooded height above the river, is the Lycée, which houses the hospital of the Wounded Allies Relief Committee. Here I was set down, and made my farewells.

A steep ascent brought me to the hospital, built round
the sides of a courtyard planted with thick-growing syc-
amores. The building is a high one, and has wards for the
wounded on three floors. Like most French Lycêes, it has
a certain sombreness of aspect; but the interior is roomy
and spacious, and the view from the windows over the
Saône, as it sweeps between hills to the terraced heights
and distant towers of Lyons, is magnificent. The hospital
has three hundred beds. There is a wing (filled at one time
by Serbian refugee children) for the sick, who are under
the charge of a French doctor. French workers also look
after the linen and housekeeping. All the rest of the work
is in the hands of the English staff.

But a new convoy had just arrived. Every one was being
overworked and terribly busy; and I felt I should have
timed my visit more conveniently. However, the Doctor
in charge and the matron gave me of their precious time,
and I was shown both the interior of the hospital and the
wooded grounds and gardens about it on the slopes of the
hill. And I had a piece of good fortune, for it so happened
that on this afternoon a colonel of the French Army was
coming to present decorations to some of the wounded.

I had seen this ceremony elsewhere; but on this occasion
the peculiar dignity of face and bearing of the aged colonel
– all about him spoke of race, and breathed of old France
– made it specially memorable. Tall and very thin, rather
frail-looking, but very erect, the colonel was escorted into
the large ward. There was a little stir, and a general saluting,
and a certain amount of standing to attention; but French
soldiers seem incapable of the inhuman and expressionless
rigidity which is the ideal of the sergeant-major at home.

The military secretary read out the names of those to be decorated.

One was to have the *Médaille Militaire,* and a number of others the *Croix de Guerre.* After the first name had been called and the soldier's 'citation' read, the colonel drew his sword and made a little speech in the name of the Republic's President to the man who had proved himself '*bon et brave soldat.*'

The words were at once ceremonious and simple. The Colonel spoke of the debt that all her loyal children owed to France; of the pride of sacrifice; of the token now given of remembrance, and its inspiration for the new generation when in its turn it was called on to do and to suffer. As I listened to his voice, clear and firm, yet touched with a fine emotion, I understood the meaning of fraternity in a nation; all casual and formal difference of age and office, rank and fortune, was drowned in the supreme and common dignity of being sons of France.

The medal was then pinned to the breast of the wounded man. On the other occasion at which I was present, the presiding General had at this moment kissed the decorated hero – a sturdy little man who had lost an eye – on both his cheeks. But, perhaps, because the soldier in this case was supine on his bed and could not raise himself, that customary salute was omitted.

I had now to visit a hospital at Nevers, which is about half-way between Lyons and Paris. On returning to my hotel – a longish journey by a succession of trams – I found that unless I was to waste a whole day, so ill-timed and infrequent were the trains, it was necessary to start the same evening and catch the express from Marseilles.

Waiting at the station I saw a group of English bluejackets hurry past, tumbling over each other with jokes and laughter, to catch a train just starting. The P.L.M. in these days is a highway of many peoples and thronged with many uniforms of many services besides the horizon-blue of the French infantry, the mustardy khaki of the Colonial troops, the dark-blue of the Chasseurs Alpins, and the medley of various uniforms, difficult to get on terms with, of the officers of the French Army. Russians with broad *épaulettes*, Serbians, occasional Italians, Belgians (I had travelled the night before with two Belgian officers on leave, one from Dixmude, the other from East Africa); an English troop-train, stopped on the line, with hundreds of cheerful soldiers in shirt-sleeves taking their ease, smoking or washing at a pump – such are common sights of the P.L.M. between Paris and the Mediterranean.

As the express was certain to be crowded, I presented myself to the *contrôleur*, who politely assured me that I should certainly have a seat. He kept his word. When the train came in I was invited to step on first of the waiting crowd, as having 'an urgent mission.' No slight advantage, for the train was soon packed, corridors and all.

Stumbling out of the train at Nevers between three and four in the morning – what with the dark stations and my own sleepiness, I was fearful of missing it – I found the platforms thronged with a multitude of soldiers, sitting or standing in a disconsolate drowsiness, or asleep on the bare stone with their packs under their heads. I wished for some magic power to transport a canteen of the *Dames Anglaises* to that dark station and open it then and there.

After knocking up one hotel in vain – all its beds were full – I found another which could take me in, and after two nights of sitting up in the crowded train was glad of a few hours' sleep.

The morning was brilliant and the air exhilarating when I drove out of the town a little way into the country, and soon found myself at the English Hospital. It is housed in a group of big, plain, modern buildings intended to be depots of the P.L.M. railway. Not picturesque, therefore, and with somewhat bare surroundings; but on the other hand the hospital has free air all about it, and has none of the many drawbacks and dirt-lodging capacities common to most old buildings. It has bathrooms and a system of heating. The French *gestionnaire*, who, I learnt, had been with the hospital from the first, took me into his office (he spoke an excellent English), and then went to find the *Médecin-chef*, a very distinguished English surgeon – famous, too, among runners in his youth; three times in succession he won the Three Miles' Race for Oxford. The wards we now went the round of were pleasant and sunny; they were full of cheerful patients, though at the moment the hospital was wanting more wounded than it could get. One fine, spacious ward contained over sixty beds. The X-Ray room leads out of the operating theatre, so that the patient could be operated on under the X-Rays in the dark, if necessary, with the least amount of inconvenience.

Everything in the hospital seemed to be admirably ordered. Things were done briskly; and one had an impression of cheerful animation both among the staff and the patients. The English nurses lodge in chalets near the building. Orderlies are supplied by the French; and French girls give their services in mending clothes and looking after the linen.

This hospital is an *Hôpital Autonome*.

Early in the afternoon I left for Paris. For the first part

of the journey the railway skirts the Loire; and one caught glimpses of that spacious stream, looped among sandy islets, and with oozy wide margins of reed-bed and poplar, and towns upon the hills beyond.

Saone and Rhone, Loire, Garonne, and Seine : how full of personality are these noble rivers, whose rich veins animate great tracts of glorious country. Their presence is felt as a felicity, even at a distance. Some involuntary prompting of the old pagan intuitive feeling about them, as of tutelar spirits or divinities, comes into the mind when one pictures these rivers of France; and I understood more nearly what France means to the simple tiller of her soil, how passionately he springs to her defence, and dies to save her.

IN THE VOSGES

'At this point,' said my companion, 'we are within four hundred yards of the German trenches.'

It seemed incredible.

We were high up on the side of the thickly wooded hill, the curves of which were followed by the road. It was an excellent road, and I was surprised to learn that it had been entirely made during the war. But what peace was in the air! A lazy, luxurious silence, with nothing but a slight warm wind trembling among the anemones and shifting ever so little the blue shadows of the pines. Yet just the other side of the ridge was the enemy. A few shells had come over that morning. But all was quiet now : and though an expert eye would doubtless have known that the sleeping, scented wood was full of cunningly hidden guns, war seemed as distant as in some valley in western England.

We had just visited a First Aid Post among the pines. Close under it were two ambulances, waiting by the dugout which was the temporary home of the drivers.

This post is one of half a dozen served by Section 5 of the British Ambulance Committee. The headquarters of the section is a little town in a valley. A number of roads radiate from this centre, which is also a railhead. There are perhaps thirty volunteers and paid drivers in the section. And each taking his turn of a spell of five days, they spend their time at one post or another. There are usually two cars at each post, each with two men. The men live in dug-outs while on duty, and their work is usually done at night, and practically always under fire. You may be sure that where a car can go, there it will be taken. But there are places where a car cannot go in the mountains, especially in the winter snows. And then Alaskan dogs with sledges are brought into service; and the motor-cycles with stretchers attached, whose splendid work has been described on an earlier page of this book.

We had reached the headquarters of Section 5 the evening before, after a long drive over the mountains.

I had come from Paris by railway with a French officer, who in the office in the Rue Pinel, now so familiar to our ambulance men, looks after the affairs of the British convoys, and makes the ways smooth for the drivers as they come and go. I had called on this officer a week before, and found him with his foot in plaster, the result of an accident; but he expressed the firm intention of accompanying me to the front, and, though I think at the cost of considerable pain, was to be my most efficient and courteous guide.

At Belfort, where we left the train, the streets glared with blazing heat. It was astonishing to hear from the B.A.C. officer and chauffeurs, who met us with a powerful car, that it was impossible to go over the Ballon d'Alsace, as had been planned, because the snow was so deep on the road. They had tried to come that way in the morning, but all their efforts had been baffled.

We had therefore to take another route. My chief regret was that this meant missing an English canteen which I had purposed and particularly wished to visit, at Bussang. The three hours' drive was one which, if the war could have been forgotten, was enchanting. It was the height of spring. Everywhere in the valleys, as we wound among them, were innumerable fruit-trees, shining with clouds of blossom; and as we gradually climbed to the higher ranges, and patches of snow appeared in clefts of rock or on the summit-slopes, we would pass grassy shoulders entirely covered with millions of blowing daffodils.

Evening was falling when we arrived at our destination, a villa beside a small lake which serves as headquarters for Section 5, and we dined pleasantly in the hospitable messroom. A French officer and *sous-officier* are attached to each section; and the conversation was now in French, now in English, which both officers had to perfection. Two men of the section were leaving to join the English Flying Corps. We drank their health, and the commander of the section made a little farewell speech, full of praises for their fine service with the convoy, their daring and devotion. I noted the terms of frank and cordial intimacy on which the French officers and the English were with each other. Much merriment passed between them; especially over a jest that they had jointly played off, the day before, on an outpost hospital on the mountains. At this hospital an *infirmiere* was expected to arrive. The head of the hospital was always playing practical jokes on the men of our convoy when they visited it, and they determined to be revenged. A young chauffeur, dressed up as a nurse, looked charmingly plausible with his fresh English complexion. He was taken up to the outpost and introduced. The hospital staff were entirely taken in, and full of gallant attentions, when a shell burst quite near. The pretended *infirmiere,* quite used to such things, moved not a muscle. There was natural astonishment, then suspicion, and the scene exploded in laughter.

In the particular sector we were to visit, no wounded have been evacuated, since the beginning of 1915, except by British ambulances.

At the point where we passed so close to the German

trenches there was, as I have said, a singular absence of any trace of war.

But during the morning, as we climbed the hills and descended the valleys, there were sufficient relics of battle and destruction, though the glory of May was over everything, and for the moment it was hard for anything to appear dead or defeated. Radiant foliage masked the ruins of farms and factories except at a close view. But nothing could disguise the broad rents in pine-woods devastated by artillery, or the gaps on the sky-line where a ridge was swept for a certain distance of everything but charred and shattered trees.

In order to visit the whole sector, we had to make long detours and return upon our tracks. Now we were in the warmth of smiling sheltered valleys, now on the heights from which one looked out far over the valley of the Rhine to the Black Forest beyond.

At a certain post on a mountain top we were warmly greeted by the staff of a little hospital which the French have installed there. It is what is called an Alpine Post; and this one is ingeniously constructed in duplicate, below ground and above. When there is a bombardment, the staff transfer themselves, and the patients are carried, under-ground, where there is an exact counterpart of the rooms above. We were pressed for time, having much to visit; but our French friends insisted on making tea, and a young officer of the famous Chasseurs Alpins, witty and gay, whether speaking his own tongue or admirable English, took me round the little hospital and showed me all its ingenious contrivances.

But there was a greater surprise in store. ' You must see our theatre,' he said. I imagined an operating theatre. But no, it was a theatre for entertainments, rigged up with stage and scenery complete.

'And if the audience is not enthusiastic, we can always rely on the shells for salvoes of applause!' In fact, as we emerged on the mountain road, though at the moment all was quiet, the mark of the enemy met the eye. A shell had struck a roofed-over recess in the rock which served as garage to one of the English cars. Happily the car was away at the time.

Great slides of snow were clinging to the mountain slopes, though, the wild spring flowers were in every crevice of earth. We descended to a hollow of the hills, cupping a black tarn, on which a sheet of ice still floated.

Here, taking gas-masks, we set out to walk. From vantage-points on the path one had wonderful views, both of the snow-streaked summits which have been the scene of such desperate fighting, and of the country below, green with many-folded valleys.

One village spire was on French territory, the next beyond on German, though there was nothing to tell this to the eye. And at times one could see the ribboned seams of the rival trenches, quite near, following irregular parallels over the undulations of the country. The desultory sound of an occasional shell lumbering over and bursting was all the sign of war.

After walking for some time in single file on an exposed slope, we suddenly plunged into a *boyau* or communication trench, roofed with boughs. It was hot and airless in the *boyau*, which seemed interminable. Now and then we met soldiers, in twos and threes, brown-faced under their blue helmets, trudging to their outposts.

At last we emerged.

It was an extraordinary scene in which to find oneself. The stony slope of a mountain-side rose before us. The trees may once have been thick upon it, though now but a ragged remnant. Over the shoulder of the hill could be seen, clear in the evening sun, a desolated summit, rustcoloured, with all its forest burnt and shot away, save scattered ragged stumps and splinters. How many brave lives had perished on those slopes! But where we stood there was every sign of industrious human animation. Infantrymen and orderlies passed to and fro.

I must not describe all I saw and was shown. But what I saw intensified my admiration of the French genius for creating order and adapting hard necessity to use.

I found that we were to dine with a French officer of the Army Medical Service. He came to meet us with a cordial greeting. The Doctor, not tall, but square and strong, with black moustache and bright observant eyes, had served for years with the army in Algeria.

A little later, as we passed along, two enemy aeroplanes came over flying at a great height in the bright evening stillness. Anti-aircraft guns at once opened on them, with quick, eager reports. White puffs appeared in the distant blue; and a tinkle of falling fragments sounded on the rock near by. The Doctor with a smile drove us in to shelter. And now an orderly announced that dinner was ready.

The dug-out, with its curved inner shell of corrugated metal, had been adorned with decorative paintings by a former occupant interested in marine zoology. It was snug, cheerful, home-like. We had an excellent dinner, admirably cooked, and seasoned with pleasant talk. We discussed national characteristics and customs; and we English tried to explain to the French doctors some of the labyrinthine strangeness of our insular character, our absurd shyness, even amongst ourselves, and the odd ways in which an Englishman disguises his emotions. We drank to the friendship and better understanding of the two nations, and I think on both sides the wish was warm. Time passed quickly, and before we were aware night had fallen.

Out in the darkness we sought the post from which an ambulance was to take back the wounded. The ambulance had already arrived. Since the road is under fire, it cannot be traversed by day, and by night only without lamps.

There were five wounded in the ambulance, and as all happened to be sitting cases, my companion and I took our places with them, after farewells to our hosts.

We began to descend the mountain-road. It is simply a succession of hairpin bends, on the corners of which the German guns are trained. Showing no light, the car felt its way down the zigzags, but the driver knew his road by heart, and our progress was surprisingly smooth and easy. Every other minute a star-shell exploded a mild radiance over the valley. We sat and talked in the darkness, and as each voice made itself heard from this corner or that – lowtoned phrases, tired exclamations, little humorous comments – the intermittent, tentative talk of casually met people – one could not help speculating on the character of the voices and wondering what sort of corresponding face would be revealed when the lights should disclose us to each other.

At last we were over the pass. Two sudden long beams of light leapt out from the lamps in front, and inside the ambulance we could be safely lit up too. There were the bandaged *Poilus*, friendly and familiar types with their brown faces and quiet eyes, comparing reminiscences in a matter-of-fact, reticent way – reminiscences of the war that already seems to have filled a lifetime.

The road by which we had come so smoothly and safely has seen terrible things, when the battle raged on the mountains for weeks at a time and the Germans burst their huge shells over the road and smothered it with splintered rocks. Our ambulances were then at work incessantly. On one side of the barrier they could only work in the darkness; on the other they worked both by day and by night, carrying the wounded down to railhead and hospital, and saving one knows not how many lives by the narrow margin that secured an early treatment.

The reader may be able to imagine just a little of what this work is like from what I have described. But winter lasts long in the Vosges, and to understand the real conditions of the service, you must picture the depth of frozen snow, the bitter cold, the slushy mire of the thaws, added to all the difficulties and dangers of the steep mountain roads, along which the ambulances must drive. I regretted that I had not been among the Vosges in the snow-time, that I might better understand. There have been casualties and deaths among the men of our various convoys with the French; but for the most part one would think, after a glimpse of their work and with a knowledge of what it means, that their lives are charmed. For my part, I found myself wondering how any of them had survived.

SOME CANTEENS IN THE WAR ZONE

We were leaving the mountains behind us; and as the car rounded the corners of the white road, the face of the country gradually changed and took on softer outlines.

I looked back regretfully to the pine-clothed ranges, wishing that time allowed us to turn back, and visit the English canteen on the distant mountain pass.

The lady in charge of this canteen has written me an account of it, from which I shall take leave to quote.

It is a canteen at a station, not very far from the front. Work begins at half-past four in the morning. The men returning to the front from their leave take the train which starts at five. But even at half-past four there are sometimes men waiting, who have walked down from the trenches. And in the long winter the snow through which they have to tramp is over their knees or even up to their chests. The men returning from leave arrive with sad looks, for they have just parted from their families; they are tired and sleepy, and though they do not grumble, they are cheered and comforted by hot coffee, a cigarette, and a word of welcome at that dreary hour of the morning.

And now to quote the *Directrice*, who, though she found the work exacting – 'when one is not providing food, one is providing conversation' – was chiefly anxious to be moved nearer the front, where there would be an opportunity for serving more men and having still harder work. 'It is all most interesting' (she wrote), 'and the more one knows the Poilu, the more one likes him.':

> Some of the soldiers insist on paying something; and when we say that all is *gratuit* they say we must

give it to the *blessés*. The older men with families are only too thankful to get a good meal for nothing, as everything costs so much now. Besides, in this part of the world so many cafes are shut, or only open for a short time daily. And many have two, or even three days' journey after they leave us, so that several francs a day mounts up.

We had a boy of nineteen the other day who asked for 'a very little *bouillon*,' and took out his purse. He was told that it was all free; and that we gave bouillon, meat, and coffee. He looked immensely relieved, and ate a large plate of bouillon and a big slice of meat; and then he confided to us that he had a long journey before him, and everything cost so much. So we 'stoked' him thoroughly before he started. He was just a hungry boy with a healthy appetite.

I explained to a man one day that all was gratuity when he had put down fifty centimes. He picked it up and then put it down again, for I told him that the Government gave the meat and coffee, and we did the cooking only. 'But why should you take all that trouble for nothing?' said he, and offered me the money. I said, ‹Monsieur, it is not for nothing, it is for the pleasure it gives us to do something for the French Army!' He looked perfectly delighted; said that was really *chic*, and resumed his money. They certainly meet all friendliness more than half-way.

Any man that speaks English, however little, always airs it. It is sometimes a little surprising, and frequently has a marked American accent. One gentleman this morning, at our 5 a.m. reception, saluted me with 'Well, Girls!' in a very American voice, as he put his quart down for some coffee. It was said in a most polite tone, which made it sound extremely funny. 'Oh, you speak English!' said I, and he beamed with satisfaction. Yesterday we had a French Hindu with an Indian detachment; a corporal, smart and intelligent. He had been in an English family in Madras; spoke excellent English, and said what a pleasure it was to hear English ladies' voices again. Many tell us they hope to come to England after the war.

A good many of our men come from the *pays envahis*. We have put up in the *foyer* of the canteen the addresses of societies helping to find or get news of *réfugiés*. It is very sad for the permissionnaires who have no home or family. Two came through the other day, who were to spend their leave in barracks in Paris. I suppose they would be the better for a change from the trenches; but it was pathetic, when all the others had somewhere to go where they were sure of a welcome. We gave them an address in Paris, where they could make inquiries for their families, of whom they had heard nothing for months; and they seemed ever so grateful for the chance of doing something definite. They felt that, after all, there was some use in having leave.

We have heard some tragic tales of the carrying into captivity of little daughters and young sisters. And as the men say gloomily : "When we get into Germany, we can do nothing to their women and children; for we are civilised."

There was a brush with the Boches a short time ago. They got them into a communication trench, and turned machine-guns on them. Few Boches, survived. One man frankly rejoiced, but was pulled up by the others for going into too many details before us. Another, a young sergeant, said it was perfectly revolting, and he had loathed the whole business, which was one of the most appalling sights he had ever seen. Though equally glad of the victory, he had not enjoyed the carnage. Probably the other man had the greater reason to hate them, and felt it was only retribution. They are very good to their prisoners. No doubt you have noticed the men with rings, with bits of glass from Rheims set like jewels in them. They are always rather grim, and mean business when they meet the enemy.

The men from the Midi find this climate little to their liking. It is a hard life anywhere of course; but two days' tramping through deep snow, even with 'leave' at the end of it, adds much to the misery of trench-life in winter. They all appreciate the canteen immensely.

What strikes one most is that they all consider themselves as such aged men after about forty-three. But there is no doubt that the life does tell very much on the older ones.

The other day we were presented with a poem written in the canteen. The men generally come in with one or two "copains" (pals), and take their bouillon in little parties at the same table. We have three rows of tables down the *foyer*. A soldier came up to me with a paper on which was written 'Miss; Misses!' He wished to know if this was the plural of 'Miss.' I said it was; and he retired to his two friends, one of

whom was the poet. Before they left they thanked
us, and presented us with these verses:

Respectueux Souvenir des Soldats du Régt. d'Inf

Vigilantes et secourables,
À qui paya l'impôt du sang,
Vous êtes toutes adorables,
Aimables Misses de Bussang.

Pour nous les permissionnaires
Vos soins affables et charmants
Paraissent les préliminaires
Du doux accueil de nos mamans.

Dans la tendresse qui nous gagne
Nous regrettons pourtant ici,
O sœurs de la Grande Bretagne!
De ne vous dire que Merci.

Puissons-nous, bien chère espe'rance,
Vous prouver en un prochain jour
Avec notre reconnaissance
Notre plus fraternel amour.

V——, Caporal,
Signaleur du 1er Bataillon – Rt.

If any one can find it in his heart to criticise verses so
full of cordial and graceful feeling, I do not envy him. But
though they do not always write in verse, the *Poilus* have
the art of expressing gratitude and friendship in a way that
shames us tongue-tied English. If I were to quote half the
letters that have come from soldiers to our workers in hos-

pitals, canteens, and convoys, I should fill many volumes.

While I was in Paris I saw a copy of a provincial paper in which the men of a certain regiment had had printed their testimony of thanks to the English canteen in their district, and it was charmingly worded.

But to return to our journey.

Early in the afternoon we arrived at the little town of Remiremont, and sought out the '*Cantine des Dames Anglaises.*' This was in the barracks; for it was a *Dépôt des Éclopés*, that is, as we have explained already, a military dépôt for tired men sent back from the front for a few weeks' rest.

This canteen was started in December 1916, and had therefore been going for five months. I found the *Directrice* and her daughter behind the counter in a room on the ground floor. They were dispensing refreshments to a group of soldiers, and at the same time helping them to piece out jig-saw puzzles, over which the men pored with the exasperated fascination that occupation provokes.

The canteen, I found, was open from eleven to twelve-thirty in the morning, and from two till five in the afternoon; but the working hours of the staff were, of course, much longer.

The Government supplies tea, coffee, and sugar; also bones and vegetables for the soup. Invalid dishes are cooked for the infirmary. Three times a week cigarettes are given out; and if there has been a victory for the Allies, French and English cigarettes are given out together; it is the kind of pleasant touch which appeals to the Poilu.

The men are terribly tired, I was told; they need rest for the mind as well as for the body. A barrack is not an exhilarating place in which to rest, though delightful enough, no doubt, after the trenches. But the presence of these Englishwomen makes a very human difference.

The soldiers soon make friends, and then they tell of their troubles, of the anxiety about those they have left at home, of all that is on their minds; we can imagine with what relief, to have womanly sympathy ready to listen! And they ask about England; it is a fresh interest to counter the dull pressure of care and monotony. 'They think it so heroic of us to have dared to cross the Channel!' the *Directrice* told me, smiling; 'to them it seems a most dangerous undertaking!' Imagination pictures the narrow seas sown thick with mines and crowded with submarines.

A point is made of always having flowers in the canteen. I noticed jars full of blossom, and saw what a brightness they made in the place. I heard that the men from the Midi have always a word and a brightening face for the flowers; it is something they have missed too long.

When the men depart, each is given a little present. They are loth enough to go, as you may guess.

Resuming our journey northward towards Nancy, we stopped an hour or so later at Rambervillers.

Here, also in the barracks outside the town, was another *Dépôt des Éclopés*, and a *Cantine des Dames Anglaises*. But we had arrived at an hour when nothing was going on but preparations by the staff. I noticed the decorations in the rooms, and the trouble spent on making the place cheerful and attractive.

As this was a canteen of the same type as the one I had just visited at Remiremont, there was nothing new to learn. Just at the moment, they told me, things happened to be very quiet.

The next canteen I visited, two days later, was at the little town of Revigny, now half battered and burnt into ruins.

Perhaps none of our canteens is kept more continually busy than the canteen at this station. We passed through Revigny in the morning, and the canteen was not open; but I saw the capable English lady who manages it, and she told me how much coffee they served out in a month; it was 280,000 cups, a figure which conjures up a little ocean of fragrant liquid. But if you have, as sometimes happens, some thou ands of men a day coming through, all tired and eager for refreshment, you have need of a running river for the relays of soon-emptied cauldrons.

The canteen is at work from one to six in the morning, often at full pressure. How I regretted that I had not been able to spend a night at the canteen and seen it in full operation!

So far the canteens visited had been either station canteens or canteens for *Dépôts des Éclopés.* There still remained the third type, the canteens for the *Dépôts des Isolés.* I saw one of these last, when I visited Troyes. In the outskirts of that old city, in the yard of a factory building, I found the canteen, and cheerful faces of the *Dames Anglaises* at the window-counter, and little knots of soldiers drinking coffee or coming for a postcard and a chat. I had a charming welcome. The first thing that caught me was the canteen's attractiveness to the eye. In the ugly yard, with its bare, sombre surroundings the canteen shed made a little island, full of hints and associations of home and women's handiwork and daintiness, with its pretty curtains, its pots of flowers, the glimpse you had of its simple gaiety of decoration.

The *Isolés* come and go, rarely staying more than a day or two. Here are lost sheep who have somehow strayed from their regiment on a journey and are waiting for it to be found for them, and other migrants on their way to or from the lines. I was introduced to the lieutenant in charge of the soldiers, who showed me over the place; the great bare room where the men have their *soupe*, at eleven in the morning and five in the evening, and over that, upstairs, an immense loft with row on row of beds of straw. It was all clean and orderly. On the other side of the yard we found the *foyer*, where men were sitting, writing letters and postcards, or reading newspapers or magazines. A piano stood in one corner. The lieutenant told me what a world of difference the canteen made, how much it lightened the appalling boredom of the war.

The canteen is open from nine in the morning till seven in the evening. Coffee is the staple refreshment. Over eleven thousand litres of it, I found, had been dispensed during the preceding month. But tea, milk, eggs, cigarettes, chocolate, air-pillows, letter-paper, postcards, and pencils are also things served out at the canteen. Seven to eight hundred a day is the average number of soldiers served. In the *foyer* the ladies of the staff get up little concerts and sing to the men. In the winter they have a cinema.

I came away, wishing to linger. Here was the best sort of work being done, and I would have liked to share in it.

VERDUN TO CHALONS

Outside Bar-le-Duc we were stopped for our papers to be scrutinised.

There, at the cross-roads, on a new signpost of bare, unpainted wood was the direction in big letters: A VERDUN. The name thrilled.

How often in those momentous days of June 1916, when the very skies, with their alternations of bright heat and cold, stormy rains, seemed to reflect the agitation of our spirits and the fluctuating crises of the battle – how often, helping carry men wounded the day before at Thiaumont or Fleury, had I tried to picture in my mind the actual aspect of Verdun and its surroundings! In those evenings we would go up on the hills that we might listen better to the noise of the guns; the sullen thudding never ceased, and intermittently came spasms of rapid shocks, and one felt the battle mounting to fury. At night, lying awake or half asleep, I would picture that endless train of cars and lorries which was driving in the darkness to and from the fortress through a rain of explosions and feeding the obstinate, superb defence.

This morning we were bound for the headquarters of more than one ambulance section in the Verdun region. Two of these sections were British Red Cross convoys. The officer in charge at headquarters – in private life known to me as a librarian in a famous library – welcomed us at Bar-le-Duc, gave us luncheon, and took us with him in the staff car on this tour of inspection. Since I happen to share with him an interest in Oriental art and history, our talk now and then rebounded from the war and from our immediate business to regions detached from Time, that seemed oddly incongruous with the scenes we were visiting. And yet at a turn of the road, here were a troop of yellow-uniformed Annamese soldiers, mending the road with Oriental industry, and looking at us as we passed with bright curiosity in their black almond eyes. The remote East had come to us here in the midst of France.

In one of the muddy and desolate hamlets of this region we found BRCS Section 17. The staff was quartered in a roomy sort of old farmhouse, with large stables which made a garage for the ambulances. The accommodation was rough, especially for volunteers of a certain age, used to the comforts of their own homes. But all had cheery faces, and gave us a good welcome. Many of the men were busy cleaning and overhauling the mechanism of their cars. Others were in the mess-room with the French officers attached to the section. As in the Vosges, one could not help being struck by the intimate and cordial relations between the French and English. It was the same with all the sections we visited this day. BRCS Section 16, which shared with Section 17 the most strenuous days of Verdun, was, we heard, *au repos*; but Section 18 (also veterans of Verdun) we came upon, after a long drive, quartered in a long wooden barrack, among the ruins of an abandoned village. On the way we had stopped for a quarter of an hour to greet the officers of Section 13, more pleasantly accommodated in a hamlet of orchards, where the trees were all in blossom. This is one of the convoys belonging to the Society of Friends, which had recently had so hard a time of it in the Champagne battle.

These sections were now serving the Verdun region. Their posts, where their dug-outs are and from which they bring down the wounded, are at various points in the ranges of hills that flank the Meuse, and make a barrier eastwards and northwards about Verdun. They have done magnificent work; some notion of it may be gathered from the brief record in an earlier chapter. The men look like veterans of war, as indeed they are.

For the moment this part of the front was quiescent. But Verdun has for the Germans the magnetism of fear as well as hope; it is a vantage-point that menaces them nearly : and it seems as if those trenched and fire-tormented hills would never regain peace. Only a few months from this day when all was lulled in quiet, the tempest was to break again – but this time on the French side – and our convoys once more were to be working day and night.

But never, I imagine, will it be as it was in 1916, from February to the end of June. The British Red Cross chauffeur drove us; and he described to me in a vivid language, racy of our northern Midlands, what the days and nights of the great defence were like; especially the nights! As we neared Verdun itself, he pointed out the many places by the roadside where the car had miraculously escaped being blown to bits. Frankly, he didn't mind saying that he didn't enjoy those trips: but the Colonel! The hotter the place was, the more the Colonel liked it, the more he was interested; he would actually stop the car to inspect the damage – 'Stop the car!' when the shells were banging and crashing all round us. 'Look there!' And the chauffeur pointed to a roof with a gaping rent in it. 'I thought we had gone to limbo, when that burst just over our heads. But we haven't been caught yet, though it's a wonder we're alive, I say.' I had a vision of the Colonel, who had been so courteous to me in Paris, enjoying his imperturbable cigarette and chatting with keen interest, while the high explosive spat up volumes of earth and stones, and made blanks of jaggedness where houses had been a second before. It is said that on the slightest excuse he would have taken his car into the smoking ruins of Douaumont itself, under the tornado of the battle. What wonder that the men of these convoys are salamanders?

We were now skirting a marshy meadow, all pitted with shell-holes, great and small. And before us rose Verdun. The little city is built upon a mound, with compactly clustered roofs and the cathedral rising over all. The twin towers told dark against scarred and scorched ranges of hills, an amphitheatre of desolation. To the naked eye, at a distance, the city does not show its wounds. But a strange silence hung over it. And as we turned in at the gates of the city under the gigantic stone walls of the Citadel, and began to pass along the streets, the sense of ruin rushed upon one. Not a house but was shattered and maimed. Shops with the familiar legends over the door – *'Boulangerie,' 'Quincaillerie,' 'Epicene,' 'Charcuterie'* – stood with parts of their interior still intact, and it seemed surprising that the brutal rents in them had not completed their demolition. But that was what made so singular an impression; the shapeless ruin – fallen ceilings, dislodged beams, crumpled walls – side by side with things that spoke so freshly of the old days of peace, of gossiping neighbours, of housewives shopping, of the good bourgeois at dominoes in the cafe – all the prosperous leisurely business and homely amenities of a French provincial town. And with all this there was the sense of callous defacement and desecrated privacy. Off one house the side had been torn at a blow. There was the interior forlornly exposed with its gay wall-paper and pieces of furniture and prints upon the wall; and over an upper floor a bedstead hung projecting and askew. It was a pitiful wreck not of a house only but of a home; and the sight set the mind suddenly wondering what had become of the population of this deserted, broken city? Where were the old men and women, where the children? The sunlight, making shadows on white walls, the rustling of chestnut and willow in the breeze along the Meuse and its canals that wind through and about the town, the peaceful reflections in the green water, the benches under the trees, the swallows, the bursts of blossom – all the spring stir of life and beauty sharpened the divorce between the absent and the present; they seemed to claim a human responsiveness, and there was nothing but ghostly silence.

Beyond the town, in the afternoon brightness, rose the encircling hills, their slopes zig-zagged with communication trenches. There was the Côte St-Michel; and beyond it, I knew, lay Fleury, and Fort de Vaux, and Douaumont; and on the northern side, beyond the first ranges, were the Mort Homme and the hill called 304; names for ever scored into the history of Europe; scenes of hideous slaughter and of indescribable valour; fought for with desperate tenacity, lost and won, and lost and yet again won, in the hugest and most fiercely protracted battle that this earth had ever seen.

We had turned for the homeward journey, leaving Verdun behind us. And soon we were on that famous 'Sacred Way,' on which that spring and early summer (the Clermont railway being usable no longer) an endless chain of automobiles streamed without intermission, in spite of bursts of dropping shells, bringing up supplies, guns, munitions, men; bringing back the wounded; saving Verdun. Those were times when the transport drivers had spells of twen-ty-four hours or more at the wheel without sleep; driving a five-ton lorry, with another five-ton weight of shells on it, each with a similar lorry just behind him and another just in front, blinded by the lights of hundreds of cars coming in the reverse direction, along gradients greasy with mud or slippery with frost.

To-day the road was solitary and silent in the windy sun-shine. But suddenly, as from nowhere, appeared by the poplars of the roadside the grey-blue figure of a Poilu. A single soldier tramping towards Verdun, with rifle slung, blue helmet on head, and his pack upon his back. How familiar a type! Swarthily sunburnt, clear-eyed, without angularity or swagger, he had an air suggesting indefinite resources, an elastic toughness, an independent intelligence. A very serious soldier, in his dusty steel-blue; yet assuredly the soldier has not supplanted and usurped the man. Alone on that famous, empty highway, he seemed the symbol and incarnation of the enduring soul of France.

Twilight was drawing on with a clouded sky, and rain had come up from the west, when at last we drew in at the Urgency Cases hospital, of 'Faux Miroir,' where we were to spend the night. Our host and guide had brought us all the way in his car, bumped mercilessly along the rough cross-country roads leading round to Revigny; and now we bade him farewell and he started back for Bar-le-Duc, very late, I fear, for dinner. We too were late. We had tumbled into festivities, and Faux Miroir was all bustle and preparation. The young Englishmen who act as orderlies in the hospital are noted for their inventive talent in the arts; they were giving an entertainment to the blesses, and the audience was already gathering. After a hasty supper, we repaired to the improvised theatre. The performance had already begun. Room was found for us to squeeze into at the sides; and what we saw was played with a zest and gaiety worthy of the most accomplished performers. It ended with a ballet of the Death of Pierrot, charming in its poetic sentiment. The applause was richly earned. I wished I had had the opportunity of asking some of the wounded, who have all too little distractions of the kind, but whose criticism would, I am sure, have been intelligent, what they thought of this performance by the young men who next morning were sweeping out the wards and attending to their wants.

It was still raining and promised to continue, when, next morning, after breakfast, the *Médecin-chef*, a Scottish surgeon from London, took me round the hospital. Faux Miroir is a fairly modern house, of nondescript architecture and of no great size. The hospital wards are big huts which have been built in the grounds. How the hospital, first established at Bar-le-Duc, was transferred to Revigny, has been described in an earlier chapter. It so happened that one scorching August day in 1915 I was driving in this region with the administrator of another hospital, and on our way to the ruins of Vassincourt we met part of the Bar-le-Duc unit with their furniture piled mountainously on a lorry, though I did not know that Faux Miroir was their destination.

Faux Miroir still shows traces of the Crown Prince's brief occupation. Just outside one of the windows is the grave of an officer, who, I was told, was one of his intimate friends. And German trenches run obliquely across the park, all overgrown now with tall grass.

In spite of cloud and rain, one could see that it was a

pleasant place for the wounded to be in. The park stretched all round with acres of verdure and clumps of wood. The wards, too, were airy and comfortable. All the patients had a smile for the chief's genial greeting.

I was struck by the good equipment of the hospital, among other things by a magnificent steriliser for disinfecting the soldiers' clothes; but most of all I was impressed by the atmosphere of expansiveness, of easy cordiality, which seemed to be reflected from the example of the Médecin chef.

Those who have seen the book about Faux Miroir, printed and illustrated by the staff, with contributions also from the wounded, will understand this atmosphere.

One of the sights of the hospital was a baby wild boar gambolling up and down in a house of wire-netting. The forests of Eastern France are full of wild boar, multiplied by the absence of shooting parties since 1914, and increased by numbers of their kind driven down from the Ardennes by the fighting. They do much damage to the crops on outlying farms. But this youthful tusker was as yet an engaging little animal.

Unfortunately our stay at Faux Miroir had to be brief; and all too soon the car was at the door. We stopped a few minutes in the village of Revigny to see the canteen, of which I have written already.

We left the car which had brought us from Revigny in the main street of a village, crowded with soldiers and with transport of every kind. The wide street formed a kind of shallow trough, with the houses on higher ground at either side, and the church at the end of it; and this rainy morning it was a mass of mire. Here we had a rendezvous with the officers of Section 10; and as we were a little early we had to wait for some time in the mud and wet before the staff car of the section arrived. The Commandant of the section and the French officer attached to it were in the car, and we were soon on our way to headquarters.

Section 10 belongs to the British Committee of the French Red Cross. It prides itself on the fact that all its men are volunteers; also on having been the first of the foreign sections to go on duty at the front beyond Verdun. But something of its doings has already been chronicled in these pages; and, as the reader of these pages knows, its share in the Verdun battles was not yet over.

We lunched with the officers in the upper room of a cottage in one of the forlorn hamlets of this district, but the quarters were cosy enough, and we were delightfully entertained. As we were chatting after the meal, the English convoy commander turned to me and said that no doubt I would like to inspect the section. Knowing nothing of the ways of generals, and of those whose habit it is to inspect, I was somewhat embarrassed, on descending, to find the whole of the section drawn up in two ranks in their helmets and accoutrements, as stalwart, weather-beaten, disciplined, and serviceable a body of men as any general could wish to see.

I suppose the ceremony of mutual salutes and presentations should have concluded with the kind of speech that personages of importance make on these occasions; but a gust of irresistible modesty in face of these English gentlemen, who for love of France and desire of service were living a life of splendid hardship and danger, overwhelmed my military manners. Even now, relieved of that involuntary importance of the inspector, I can but lamely express the admiration so warmly felt for these my countrymen, and the envy of all they were able to do and undergo.

Formalities over, there was opportunity for friendly talk, and, so it chanced, for renewing some old acquaintances, as we were shown the long shed where the men had their bunks and living quarters.

But we had far to go; and, after cordial farewell of the chief and his men, we were soon speeding along the road which passes the southern end of the Argonne.

That long ridge which heaves itself so strangely out of the plain, muffled with close forests – the barrier that proved so impenetrable to the obstinate thrusts of the Crown Prince in his endeavour to join up with the German armies farther south – appeared before us. It stretched away into the distance, heavily green under the dismal sky, inscrutable with its dense wood, and as if jealous of its secrets. We passed through half-ruined deserted little towns, with the rain blowing on defaced church towers and calcined walls and gaping house-fronts.

The landscape, so fresh with wounds of war, was steeped also in history. There on the eastern side of the Argonne, where the high-road threads its forest, was Varennes; and in the plain, on towards Paris, was Valmy. The place where the old France of the Monarchy yielded up its spirit; the place where the new France of the Republic rose to its feet amid the salvoes of its first victorious guns. Here, fifteen centuries ago, Attila's wild Mongol armies, overrunning Europe from the East, were stopped and shattered; here the invading Prussians, gathered to avenge the cause of all the autocrats, were rolled back by Dumouriez' ragged troops; and here the power of France was to have been broken for ever, three summers ago, by the greatest army ever known; but destiny once again was on her side. To be fighting in

Champagne is in itself an inspiration to the French soldier, conscious of that wonderful past.

Our road was now roughly parallel to the Front, which here is on a line from east to west. The villages we passed through were all full of soldiers coming and going in their muddy uniform, and of all the varied traffic that goes on behind the lines. In a big barn were assembled a battalion fresh from the trenches and preparing for rest; and some of them were singing songs and making merry. But for the most part the soldiers wore an air of grave endurance and determination. And truly the sodden roads and dripping clouds were not responsive to hilarity.

In one of these villages we found Section 20, the Scottish Red Cross convoy of the *Comité Britannique*, and in another Section 3 of the British Ambulance Committee. The officers of each of these sections gave us a good welcome, and we were shown their quarters, and had a talk of what was doing. After recent great exertions they were enjoying a comparative rest. But Section 20 was saddened by the loss of one of their members, the latest joined and youngest, in the battle of Champagne the month before. His death has been described on an earlier page. And another member, of equal youth, had died in hospital.

I should have liked to linger and see more of what these sections were doing, and the posts they served; but it was only possible to visit the posts at night, and we were due at Châlons that evening.

It was already late in the afternoon when we took farewell of Section 3, which was so good as to send us on in another car.

The last part of our journey was over the famous Plain of Châlons, that unfertile, vast, melancholy region, to which the rain and the fading of the day gave a heightened spirit of emptiness and desolation. It matched with thoughts of that unending war of the trenches manned with men so brave in disillusion, among the hills in the cloudy distance. And, suddenly, there returned to my memory, like an incarnate spirit of the soil, the figure of the solitary soldier on the road above Verdun.

IN THE MIDI

In Normandy, but a few days ago, spring was still shy and winter's long bareness timidly disputed by the first leaves, which so suddenly were to burst out in triumph. In the valleys and uplands of the Vosges it was a world of blossom. And now as the train sped along the Rhone valley, past Avignon and Aries, the hay was being carted, and fruit-pickers were busy among the cherry-trees.

I reached Mentone, my journey's end, in a rainy twilight. Grey clouds drooped over the mountains, and the sea was leaden. But early next morning, as I walked up the garden walks of *Hôpital* No. 222, the coast looked radiant and the Mediterranean had recovered its own blue.

Swinburne in one of his letters entertainingly finds an excuse for the sourness and arrogance of Carlyle's reminiscences in the fact that they were mostly written at Mentone: 'No temper, no character could be expected to remain tolerable under the influence of that hateful hole.' No doubt the vehement poet was expressing his genuine feeling. This luxurious landscape and tideless sea were alien to his physical fibre. He craved for movement in wind and water, for salt and sting. But wounded and sick men in the first weakness of convalescence feel otherwise. And Southerners, born to the sun, how they love it in their bones! How dolefully they miss its absence!

The vast hospital, once the Hotel Imperial, in which its administrator received me, seemed full of sunlit air. As we went through the spacious rooms and broad corridors, where the patients could sit at long tables for their meals; as we inspected a kitchen obviously adequate to the most royal of peace-time banquets, the store-rooms with their ample cupboards, the magnificent X-Ray installation, the *ouvroir*, the pharmacy, the baths of divers sorts, the labyrinthine resources of a modern hotel – my thoughts went back to some of the other hospitals I knew, where electricity was remote as the pole, where hot water could only be procured by boiling it on a stove, where tables and cupboards had to be improvised on the spot, where every man became a kind of Crusoe and invention was put to all conceivable tests, where dust and dirt were old and jealous inhabitants, only to be driven out by sleepless warfare.

It must be a delight to have all this smooth convenience at one's service. And yet I doubt, were it not for the sake of the patients, if the Red Cross worker in one of those other hospitals would so willingly exchange the extra labour, the endless little difficulties which have daily to be overcome, for the amplitude, the sumptuous appointments and contrivances of a modern hotel: for are not all the roughness and improvisation part of a victory achieved – the spice and savour of service?

Hospital No. 222 has five hundred beds, and its maintenance is a big affair. The question of supplies, and especially of fuel, now so scarce, is by no means an easy one. But I carried away an impression of detailed efficiency and harmonious control which had their reflection in the contented faces and manner of the patients.

Earlier in the war the hospitals of this region were filled with wounded from the Western front. But since a certain date they have been devoted to cases from Salonika. And these are suffering less often from wounds than from sickness, malarial for the most part.

On this southern coast, the sun is a great physician. You

may have all the appointments of the costliest hotel, but you cannot buy sun-baths anywhere. Here they are to be had for nothing; and the healing virtues of radiant sun are put to wonderful use.

At the little English hospital on Mont Boron, overlooking Nice, which I was next to visit, there were the same pleasant conditions, the same sensation of cleansing sunshine, and how wonderful a prospect over coast and sea! Trains being impossibly rare, I took the tram, which is slower, but a great deal more agreeable than the railway, since it climbs the heights above the sea-board, and gives an endlessly changing view of the landscape with all its blossoming profusion. One changes at Monte Carlo, and I had an hour of waiting in the trimly swept terraces and gardens of the Casino.

How this coast smells of riches!

To eyes fresh from the ruined homes of Eastern France, from the ghastly desolations and sublime endurances of the Front, this previous world of moneyed idleness, these innumerable villas perched on the hills and clouded with flowers, these glowing white walls and basking blue bays, the crowd of monstrous hotels, parasites of that glaring gamblers' Paradise in the middle of them – all seemed a transplantation from another planet, a projection of dreams into the sunlight. This was not France; it was some cosmopolitan country, detached from reality and now in some way inexpressibly exposed and forlorn, as if inhabited by ghosts of purposeless rich people driven in phantom automobiles on endless circles. Even the landscape appeared still to have an obsequious and subservient air. The red-roofed, white-walled trimness of towns and villages, the scenic heights, the soft curves of coast, the anchored yachts, the immobile blue of the Mediterranean; it was like a box of toys set out with glittering and the most expensive neatness – for whom?

Yet to the senses it was all warmly alluring. And recalling long days of illness, and slow, feeble convalescence, I tried to think myself into the state of the sick and wounded in the hospitals, and felt that just this isolation from the actual, this touch of dream, was a potent charm to conspire with Nature's instinct for recovery. I thought that to come from malarial trenches and the brutal monotony of war to this world that breathed of sun and the idle flowers might bring one whole sooner than all medicines.

My journey to Mont Boron was beguiled by interesting talk with a fellow-traveller, a French lady, who, seeing my uniform, and speaking admirable English, asked for news of England. She had a son who lived in England and was fighting with our army, and she herself had nursed our soldiers and interpreted for our officers at the battle of the Marne. She described in the most vivid manner how she had seen the triumphant Germans passing through the village where she happened to be; how they had all but shot her, because they thought she was English; how she had been taken before the General in his headquarters – none other than the famous von Kluck; how at a certain moment an atmosphere of telegrams and anxiety superseded the cocksure confidence of the advance on Paris; how a regiment suddenly appeared, retreating, tattered, bloodstained; the abrupt vanishing of the German host; and then, after a little interval, the first arrival of the English, dead-tired and mortally hungry, with a colonel at their head who was sorely put out because, though he perpetually asked for 'oofs,' he could make no one understand. You may imagine he was ready to fall on the neck of any one who could order a meal and interpret the wants of his men.

Here was an opening to expand on the deplorable lack of languages in the British Army. But my generous acquaintance, on the contrary, was only eloquent of the virtues of our countrymen at war, and became enthusiastic about the merits of English nursing. It was quite homelike to listen to this Frenchwoman, so severe on French deficiencies, so glowing in praise of England. Perhaps in long visits to our island she had acquired some of our national habits; we are all so used to this strain at home, in the complementary sense. There were so many incidents to recount, both tragic and entertaining, that we had almost slipped by my destination before I was aware of it; and I was obliged to descend from the tram with some abruptness, loth to lose the end of a story, and say farewell.

Mont Boron, rising steeply from the seashore, looks out far over Nice and its harbour to the shining Mediterranean and the beautiful sharp ridges of the Esterel in the west. High up on its seaward slope are the white buildings of the Queen Victoria Memorial Hospital. It has been explained in an earlier chapter how this hospital, which existed before the war for the needs of British patients on the Riviera, was made over at the beginning of the war to the use of the French Government, and has been filled with wounded from the French armies.

For a period of a few months during the war it was closed, but was then asked by the French Government to reopen, and promised a regular supply of sixty patients. The Directress, who held her post before war began, showed me the hospital. There was an inviting air of semi-privacy in the small, spotless wards, opening on to terraces which held the southern sun, and yet were fanned by the sea breezes and looked out into limitless space. On these terraces sat loungingly little groups of soldiers, playing games or looking on at the players, or enjoying a simplicity of basking idleness. Among them were sinewy black Senegalese, who looked up with great childish smiles of welcome. Most negroes look as if the suns of Time, through countless generations, had burnt them to a hue that has richly deepened the brown skin to their particular shade of bronze or ebony. But the Senegalese have a singular tinge of blue in their duskiness. You might fancy that they had been dipped in inky fluid, a factitious dye upon their native brownness. A certain want of familiarity with such things as chairs and tables embarrasses their movements, which are apt to be huge and sudden, so that, as I was told, the furniture was always coming to pieces under the stress of their cheerfulness. I recalled a story told in his book by Mr. Baerlein, who was with our ambulances in the Vosges, of a Senegalese found wandering stark naked by a corporal, who proceeded to arrest him. 'But it is all right,' said the Senegalese, 'we have had leave to go out in *mufti*.'

With the blacks were sundry Moors, and Frenchmen of the Midi speaking with a strong southern accent. All were native lovers of the sun; and it was good to see them responding to that congenial warmth and light, the absence of which in grey northern skies is a kind of starvation to such natures.

The hospital has an annexe at the back, higher up on the steep slope, and reached by climbing garden paths, where figures of picturesque convalescents were slowly sauntering. It is divided into four pavilions, isolated from each other, for infectious cases, if necessary, and has its own independent kitchens, offices, and nurses' rooms. Beyond this annexe are woods stretching up to the forest road of Mont Boron. These woods have been leased from the Government; and delicious shady paths, with seats, have been made among the trees.

Early next morning, having reached Cannes by an evening train from Nice, I was walking along the famous esplanade with its unshady palm-trees, and presented myself to the Director of the South African Ambulance, occupying the Hôtel Beau-Rivage, which, with its garden, fronts the sea.

Though not (so I was told) absolutely of the most modern, this hotel, like that at Mentone, makes a sumptuous hospital. You enter a spacious hall, high as the roof, with balconies on each of the four floors surrounding it. The hospital contains 225 beds, and all, as it happened, were occupied. Here again were great numbers of malarial cases.

Among the staff of our hospitals in France one is always meeting nurses, and doctors too, from Canada, Australia, and other of the Dominions overseas. But here was a whole splendid hospital equipped and maintained by South Africa. Love of France has indeed called helpers to her service from all quarters of the world. And this hospital is specially fortunate in having at its head the present Director and his wife, who, though South Africa is their home, are French themselves in blood. They are well acquainted therefore with both French and English ways, and able to interpret one to the other. Some of the wounded who have been nursed here have been touched more than a little by the thought that not only Britain but her distant dominions have sent aid to their country in its hour of need and danger; and this particular gift of a hospital so magnificent and complete is thrice appreciated because it is in the charge of representatives so sympathetic.

After going the round of the three different floors where the wounded are, and seeing the big *ouvroir* (where bandages and dressings were being made, and the clothes of the wounded repaired), the two operating theatres – one for septic operations – the pharmacy, and so on, I was taken down to the basement. It is there that the wounded are brought when they first come in. There they are stripped, helped to the bathroom and washed, and taken by lift and stretcher to their wards.

At the Beau-Rivage, as at Mentone and Nice, the sun is called in to aid the surgeon. When a man has undergone an operation, and has recovered from its first effects, he is taken out on a balcony on a fine day; all his bandages are removed, and the wound or amputated stump is exposed to the direct rays of the sun. It is astonishing how rapidly even extremely foul wounds clear up under this treatment. The sun hurries on the healing processes of nature; the wounds lose their septic appearance; and it becomes possible to close a huge gap by surgical means and obtain the same results as in a clean aseptic surface. The treatment is used of course in hospitals in the interior, but radiant sunlight is the special fortune of the Riviera.

Besides the wounded, many are the civil patients, both male and female, who are treated in the hospital, for the reputation of its surgery has spread over the district. The Director visits the civil patients in their homes as often as is necessary after the operation. The Mayor of Cannes has lent a motor car specially for this purpose. And so highly appreciated is the Colonel's work, that he has been asked by the *Service de Santé* to form a mobile unit – *Équipe de Chirurgie Volante* – for the Fifteenth *Région*. This means providing a motor ambulance with surgeons, assistants, and outfit, ready to travel in the district and perform the major operations in the civil hospitals. Such an invitation is an honour rarely offered, as may be imagined, to foreigners.

The same morning I took a fly, and drove out of the town by leafy lanes up the gentle slopes of the hills to the Villa Félicie. This is the sanatorium attached to the South African Ambulance. Tuberculous cases in an early stage, or cases where tuberculosis is threatened, are treated here; and the villa is admirably adapted for its purpose. It stands among beautiful grounds, with sloping gardens and sunny terraces. The uses of fresh air and the virtue of scrupulous cleanliness are taught in a winning and persuasive manner. The windows are kept open day and night. If a patient should break this rule he gets no dessert with his dinner next day. Such formidable punishment is very effective. The Captain and his wife, who are in charge of the hospital, gave me a charming welcome, and showed me every corner of the villa. There was a pleasant family air about it all. I was particularly struck with a group of Serbians, the first I had seen. The Captain told me they were all peasants, but had quickly learnt to talk French. They were very cleanly, he said; and they looked intelligent and good-natured. But, of course, the patients are French soldiers for the most part. The long exposure in the trenches has brought tuberculosis all too often in its train : and such an excellent sanatorium as this does much-needed work.

On my way back to Cannes, I called at the Hôtel Gallia, now a big French military hospital. I wished to have a talk with some English nurses who, I knew, had been working in this hospital since the beginning of the war. The hotel is a huge flamboyant building – German, I believe; certainly the decorations, so determined to be imposing at all costs, smacked of Teutonic taste. After being led through many corridors and a vast hall crowded with soldiers at their dinner, I at last found one of the two trained English nurses whom I sought. Her companion happened to be ill and in bed. I think it has already been explained that, apart from English hospitals for the French wounded, there are numbers of English trained nurses working in French hospitals. Their position has, from the nature of the case, not been an easy one, as they have no authority and have to fit into a system to which they are not accustomed. They also have many prejudices to contend against. The nurse I talked with has no official title or status at the Gallia; but, as I heard, she and her colleague have won by patience, tact, and the proof of skill and devotion, the esteem of the staff and the affection of the wounded. She told me that, in spite of all difficulties, she was happy in her work, and especially happy in having won appreciation of trained English nursing from the French authorities. She was now in charge of the operating theatre, and had succeeded in substituting scrupulous order and method for the more casual and nonchalant ways of the usual military hospital.

Our admiration must go out to such workers as these, scattered over France, lavishing their trained skill and experience on the care of the French wounded, for love of their own calling and of France. In paying homage to this nurse's work, we pay homage to a devoted band whose labours should not be unknown because they are wholly unadvertised.

The two trained nurses at the Gallia are assisted by a number of VADs – some fourteen or fifteen – nearly all of whom are Canadian ladies of position. These not only give their personal services, but have helped with gifts of their own and of their friends in Canada. Help has also come from the *Comité Britannique*, and I found that all 'extras' in the way of surgical instruments, etc., came from England.

My plan was now to visit Château St-Rome, near Toulouse, on my way back to Paris. The only express left Cannes in the morning about eleven. But in these days it is one thing to decide on a train, and another to travel by it. I was told that it was necessary to reserve a seat at least eight days beforehand. In the early spring three weeks or a month's notice had been required. I had no seat reserved when I repaired to the station next morning, and must take my chance. The long train drew in. At once a conductor appeared on the steps of each car and barred all passage to the besieging groups of would-be travellers, mostly officers on leave. The train was absolutely full; not a seat was vacant. Moreover, it was forbidden to stand in the corridor. I tried my best persuasion, but in vain. I demanded the *Chef de la Gare*, and explained the urgency of my mission. My status and importance rose with every minute as the train's departure approached; at the warning whistle I scaled the giddiest heights of dignity; and at last, tired by importunity, he told me that I might board either of the first two cars. My triumph was rudely dashed. 'What has the station-master to do with it?' cried the conductors. '*On ne monte pas.*' And each looked more ferocious and incorruptible than the other. The train was about to start; the disappointed travellers were falling back, resigned to the prospect of the crawling 'omnibus'; but I had a feeling that I should go in that train, and clung on to the last. Obstinacy was rewarded. Just as the wheels began to move, a young French officer at the window of the car called out to me: 'There is a vacant seat!' I hopped up past the surly conductor, and the train moved out.

Needless to say, in a few minutes the owner of the seat – another officer – appeared to claim it. It was not vacant after all. But I was to leave the train at Tarascon in the afternoon, and meanwhile there was the corridor and the restaurant, though the owner of the seat was most amiable and assured me it was quite at my disposition. The officer who had rescued me from the threatened prospect of spending a full week at Cannes, attempting each day to insert myself into an impregnable express, began now to converse in perfect English, and proved to be a professor of French in a Welsh University, when wars were not claiming him for France. He was engaged in translating Bernard Shaw's *You Never Can Tell*, which diverted the leisure of his dug-out at the front. We lunched together, talked of books, and drank to each other's country. I was sorry when the time came to part, and the train drew up at Tarascon.

Here the station was thronged with soldiers from the front in frayed and soiled blue tunics, and with others returning. But Tarascon itself seemed far enough from the trenches and from Kaiserdom.

A hundred swallows were darting and skimming in low flight over the broad and rapid Rhone. Sunset shone down the tree-bordered stream that swept eddying away into the South; it warmed the old walls and roofs of Tarascon and the huge square tower that stands magnificent and forbidding by the river, the tower of Rene of Anjou. And I thought of that old king, and his ironical destiny. Lover of all the arts and Muses, to him warfare was a stupid waste of glorious energies; but from boyhood he was always being bequeathed by thoughtless kinsfolk some distant

kingdom or estate – always in the hands of someone else
– and honour compelled him to go forth and claim it by
force of arms. Fate also gave him a terrible daughter, our
own Queen Margaret, to plague his old age with her fierce
ambitions and her scorn for his simple joys. How much of
mankind is in Rene's case to-day!

With night falling over the darkening green of the
immense fruitful plain, the train kept on through Nimes
and other cities of the South, which it was tantalising to
pass through in such haste. In the grey of the night, I
had a ghost-like glimpse of the tremendous ramparts of
Carcassonne.

Early dawn found me wandering the silent streets of Toulouse. I had some hours to wait for a train, and sought out
St-Servin's famous church, the ruddy bricks of its tower
just catching the first light of the sun; and, as I stood there
in the shadowy solitude, heard a clatter on the cobbles, and
coming past the great Romanesque apse saw one of those
incongruous apparitions of the war – a party of Annamese
soldiers, going out to work. No one else was in sight. It was
a strange juxtaposition of Oriental humanity and Western
architecture of the Middle Ages.

By nine o'clock I was driving from the station of Ville-
nouvelle. In the bright morning sunshine the snows of
the Pyrenees shone on the horizon. The day was already
hot. In a few minutes we were at the Chateau St-Rome,
the home of the *Présidente* of the *Comité Britannique* and
her husband.

The English doctor in charge of the hospital, who received
me, was wearing a French uniform and has a commission
in the French army. He has French officers for colleagues,
one of whom is the *Médecin-chef* and has charge of the

malades, and an English – or rather Canadian – assistant. The constitution of the hospital is therefore a little different from that of any of those I had visited.

The matron is a fully trained nurse; the rest of the nursing is done by English VADs. There are about three hundred beds, and nearly all happened to be full. The orderlies are Annamese.

The wounded are disposed of in various buildings in the grounds of the château. One is a large building in Renaissance style, with a *loggia*. All about is the park, with winding, shady walks. I asked if the heat were not very trying in the full summer. But the doctor told me that though the heat was sometimes intense – it was decidedly hot this day of my visit – yet the nights were cool, and there was nearly always a draught of wind along the valley of the Garonne.

At St-Rome, many of the patients must make a long stay, for since convoys of wounded ceased to come from the front, the hospital has specialised in bone-surgery and the treatment of cases where compound fractures have failed to heal. These cases – all too frequent in the war, owing usually to too hurried surgery at the outset, when the doctors were driven at high pressure – are obstinate, and demand long treatment. It must be a boon at least to find such pleasant quarters as St-Rome.

A leisurely inspection of the hospital occupied the morning. I met the genial French officers at luncheon, and one of them accompanied me to the station.

Returning to Toulouse, I took the evening train for Paris. There was the usual crowd; and before we started the corridor was packed with officers and soldiers, who slept somewhere on the floor. It was an opportunity for noticing once more the charming relations between officers and men in the French army. A Poilu would come up and ask '*mon lieutenant*' for help; he had a cross-country journey to make, and was quite at a loss; and the lieutenant would take out his time-tables and look up trains and explain the connections. There were others who sought advice on other points, and all were sure of friendly help and counsel. There was respect on one side, courtesy and patience on the other. And with it all a simple human kindness.

A MATERNITY HOSPITAL

An incident recorded by an English lady working in a canteen for the British Army in France has stuck in my mind.

A battalion of miners, if I remember rightly, had passed through the station to which the canteen was attached, and had solemnly eaten and drunken with great satisfaction, and then trooped out without a word. The ladies of the canteen were surprised and just a little hurt that no one of them said 'Thank you!' But after a few minutes an envoy – a man of another regiment – appeared, sent by the battalion to express their gratitude for them. Conscious of rough speech and ways, and feeling that they could not frame their thanks in any words which they could suppose appropriate to the ears of ladies, they had chosen this indirect shy way of showing their gratitude.

There is something touching and human in this little story; something very English too. It is certainly difficult to imagine a Frenchman, of whatever class or training, failing to find the right words in such a case. But then it is an essential part of education in France to teach the expression of thoughts and feeling in fit and clear language. How many Englishmen are taught anything of the kind?

All our workers in France know with what grace and point the wounded soldiers express themselves. There are thousands of letters which I might have quoted in this book, each delightful in form and feeling (even when eccentric in orthography and grammar), though naturally of a sameness of subject-matter. Here, for once, I cannot resist reproducing a letter from a gunner fighting in the Argonne to the Directress of the Society of Friends' Maternity Hospital at Châlons:

> *Madame la Directrice, – Veuillez avoir la bonté d'excuser la liberté que je prends de vous écrire, e'en est du reste pour moi un plaisir, et surtout un devoir. La présente est pour vous remercier du grand service que vous venez de nous rendre et de tous les bons soins que vous avez prodigués a ma femme, Mme. D——.*
>
> *C'est pour moi un puissant reconfort de relire les lettres que ma femme m'a envoyées, tandis qu'elle était votre pensionnaire, elles sont toutes à votre éloge et, grâce a vous, alors que nous sommes séparés, ma femme et moi, du fait de la guerre, j'avais la certitude que rien ne lui manquait, et qu'elle a été aussi bien soignée que l'on pourrait le désirer.*
>
> *C'est pour moi un double plaisir de penser que ma fille a vu le jour entre vos mains, et, plus tard, quand elle pourra comprendre, elle sera aussi heureuse et fière de penser à vous et à votre belle nation que j'admire et qui nous est encore plus chère pour ce que nous vous devons.*
>
> *Vous voudrez bien avoir la bonté de remercier pour moi vos infirmières qui ont été si gentilles et si dévouées pour nous, jamais nous n'oublierons tous vos bienfaits et nous penserons toujours a vous.*
>
> *En l'attente de jours meilleurs qui viendront par suite de la victoire que nous gagnerons à côté de nos camarades anglais, je vous prie, Mme. la Directrice, de croire à notre considération et à nos plus sincéres remercîments. – Votre respectueux,*
>
> Gaston D——

What instinctive courtesy there is here, not only in the

phrasing but in the thought! There are letters by other husbands, which I could quote, very far from perfect in spelling and grammar, but still so expressive, so natural in their courteous gratitude.

The little hospital occupies one wing of a large block of buildings used to house homeless old people of the Department of the Marne. On the first floor are two long wards, containing twenty-eight beds in all. On the ground floor is the *crèche*, to which the mothers may bring their older children when they cannot otherwise be cared for; it consists of two dormitories, one for boys and one for girls, and a dining-room where they can play when it is wet. The mothers remain for three weeks after the baby is born, sometimes longer; and when they leave they receive the clothing necessary for themselves, their children, and the newest baby, from the stores in England. They are visited whenever possible after they leave; for the Directress told me that she and her colleagues are above all things anxious to keep in touch with them, and make the friendship of the Friends a real and lasting thing.

These women had been fetched in an ambulance from Rheims and the villages of the neighbourhood, often under a heavy bombardment; and the devotion and courage of the staff of the hospital, who were at their exacting and dangerous work for days and nights together when the bombardment was at its worst, shine beyond all words. The month before my visit had been, in fact, an overwhelmingly arduous time.

As I went through the wards, I felt that this was indeed a haven of reassuring peace, after the places from which the women had come. As one mother says: '*Ce n'est pas gai de rester dans les caves avec les petits enfants,*' especially when you have no cellar of your own and have to share a neighbour's. Earlier in the war it was not so much from bombardment and the misery of a cellar life that the patients had suffered, as from exposure and privation. The breadwinner was gone; all the doctors had been mobilised for the campaign; and the houses were scarcely habitable. It was in those earlier days (the Directress has recorded) that an expectant mother was 'brought away from a small shed, about twelve by fourteen feet, the only lighting other than the door being a piece of glass a foot or so square let into the planking.' On a pile of straw on the earthen floor slept three men, four women, and six children! 'Here, two months before we came, a baby had been born. The mud was six inches deep before the door, but, in spite of this and of our unexpected visit, the six children were all clean, and on a string across that wretched hovel were hanging a few meagre articles of children's clothing, not only washed but ironed!'

What a fine self-respect, through every degradation of circumstance, is seen in that brief glimpse! The hospital was nearly full on the morning of my visit. In one of the wards a woman, whose house had been burnt over her head only a week before – she came from one of the bombarded villages – lay between her twin infants of a few days old. Tiny creatures, with faces as of sages wrinkled with disgust at this miserable world, they were in that ruddy stage of babyhood which is apt to awe rather than charm the igno-rant male, even though he be the father. But mothers are wiser. They do not wait till the mysterious transformation of infancy replaces those rueful puckers with flower-like bloom; they even regret perhaps each day that, familiarising the baby with the interest of its new world, removes its helplessness a little further from the first thrilling maternal intimacy. The mother, dark-haired, and with dark eyes large in the pallor of her face, brought a smile from the depths of her great weariness. She looked from side to side, and she seemed content. She had the look of one who knows that all cares for the time being are lifted from her. Yet it was the face of one who had passed through immense pain.

Downstairs were the children. Some tiny still; others of three or four years; others of yet greater age and experience. They had toys to play with; they played, or talked, or slept in their cots. There was a happy air in that room. Georges and Georgette, Pierre and Susanne, how much will you remember, I wonder, of this strange and terrible world you happened into and which you take so calmly in these sheltering walls, where instead of father and mother the *Demoiselles Anglaises* feed you, and medicine your ailments, and play with you, and kindly scold you when you forget their orders, and tuck you up at night?

Some of the children were getting rosy cheeks and a plumpness of round limbs, but some were still pale with the pallor of the cellars from which they came. For in the perpetually bombarded city and the little towns and villages in its neighbourhood there are thousands who live perforce an underground life. And the children, starved of sun and air, grow white with the unnatural whiteness of a mushroom in the dark cellars.

It is only with pangs and reluctance that a French mother gives up her child to another's custody, even in such circumstances. But the mothers give their children to the *Demoiselles Anglaises*, if tearfully, yet without misgiving. For the word has gone about that these are indeed friends in trouble; they know whom they may trust.

I saw in the garden a kind of wooden shelter, airy as possible, in which were slung a number of little cots and hammocks, where the sunshine and the fresh air – fetish of les Anglais as the French are apt to think it – do marvels with those pale young cheeks.

It was on this same day that I watched the battlefield, sinister with all the science of desolation, and heard the guns blankly echo about the flayed and barren hills. Barrenness and destruction triumphed there, as if men's one desire were to disnature earth, to blast the tree, choke the spring, shrivel the grass, and most of all to break, maim, blind, and utterly destroy the body into which their souls were born. But here, snatched from desolation, shielded and cherished, life was budding and flowering; restorative nature sought its old channels. To look on these sleeping faces of infancy, to watch the young movements of the children in their play, made the distant thudding of the guns seem unreal, or at least a transitory terror and destined to defeat.

There, was nothing but ends; here, all was beginning. There, was shattering mechanism; here, was growing life.

I seemed to see, out of all this blood, and all these tears, young France re-risen.

A THOUGHT FOR THE FUTURE

The reader has now some idea of the scope of the work that Britain has done in aid of the wounded and the war victims of France. It is right that this work should be known, and this country may well take pride in it as good service loyally rendered. But it has been essentially a labour of love. It has been as the gift of friend to friend; and our chief pride and satisfaction is that France has accepted this token of friendship and allowed us the privilege of taking some small part in the caring for her wounds.

For we must not exaggerate. Let not any reader of this little record forget for a moment how vast has been the burden which France has borne and is bearing. The help that we have been able to give to her wounded and sick has been generously appreciated by the French, and in actual amount is not inconsiderable. Yet in a comprehensive view of the whole work of the *Service de Santé* and the Red Cross in France it may seem small enough, statistically measured. It is only when we view it in a larger light and in the purely human aspect, that this voluntary labour of British men and women assumes a deeper value and significance. It is not so much work carried through as seed sown in the future. That the friendship between England and France should be firm, loyal, and enduring; that it should be rooted in reality and knit by mutual understanding as well as esteem; this is a matter of supreme moment for the future of Europe. And for the furthering of that good end may it not be that the work described in these pages will have done more than speeches of statesmen or commercial treaties, perhaps more than any other agency?

Nothing has been more vividly proved by the world's experience in the war than the shallowness of the calculation that nations are governed solely by self-interest and fear. At bottom what one nation feels for another is of the same stuff and the same inspiration as what one man feels for another man. In the end we come down to human issues. Truly the preservation of oneself is the sovereign motive of action; but that ' self,' of what splendid, as well as ignoble, things it may be compounded! And to save its integrity how many have given up possessions, home, happiness, existence! The action of Belgium, the action of the British Dominions, the action of the United States – these reveal what human nature is, they are events to make us 'feel that we are greater than we know.'

What does a man stand for? Of what fibre is he made? What choice does our instinct tell us that he will make in a crisis? Is he one whom we cannot help loving, and doing sacrifices for, in spite even, it may be, of fault and weakness? So we judge of men, or feel about them in ways beyond judgment and reason, and so we act in their regard. But it is essential that we should know them as persons, by personal contact and experience.

The trouble is that between nations there is so little opportunity of real acquaintance. Mists of ignorance float between them and solidify into walls of prejudice. Governments misinterpret the people they govern. And the old primeval instinct of dislike for the foreigner, simply because he is different and strange, survives and is not easily dislodged.

When after the few days of anxious suspense it was known that England was to take her stand by the side of France, there was a recoil of profound relief. With this satisfaction at the prospect of strong support in a struggle of which the terrible character was far more clearly realised in France from the first than in this country, there was mingled a warm appreciation of England's loyalty. The power and vast resources of our Empire were known, even perhaps exaggerated in the popular mind. But the difficulty of bringing this enormous power readily into action was not understood. As a French writer has told us, when the length of the British front was first announced, there was a feeling of blank disillusion. The old distrust of English policy made itself heard here and there. There were those who thought, what the Germans wished them to think, that England would let France do all the fighting, and then step in for the spoils. Instructed opinion knew better, and could appreciate at something like its true value the services of our Navy. But it was natural that those who had but a vague notion of Britain as a world-wide empire, should contrast that fraction of the front which our army held with the immense line held by the French, and ask why so great a power was doing so little. Then came the report of our new millions of soldiers. Great camps arose in France. And still, among a people used to military service as a part of national life, it was asked, what these millions were doing, and why were they not in the firing-line beside the French whose manhood was being drained of its best blood. 'We will go through with you to the end,' Kitchener had said, 'but you must have patience and give us time to prepare.' Patience is hard in the midst of a mortal struggle. The marvellous speed with which our improvised armies were trained seemed like slowness.

At last came the battles of the Somme. The quality of our new armies shone out before the world, and the French, ever quick to admire, began to understand the magnitude of our effort and achievement. That understanding has been steadily and surely growing with our increasing efforts, and with each new blow that our armies have struck. Our inevitable first delay may still be lamented; the weight of our aid is no longer belittled.

And what of the English people? What did they think of the French? It must be said that before the war our country-people knew very little of their nearest neighbours. Far less than in some former times. After the war we may hope that the intellectual and social relations between the two countries may recover that old and mutually invigorating closeness of intercourse that prevailed in the eighteenth century among the educated classes of a far smaller population. But though for a number of decades the general ignorance of France and the French among the people of Britain had perhaps rather increased than diminished, yet there was a certain traditional sentiment about France among us that has never been extinguished. Philip Sidney's famous phrase in one of his sonnets, 'our sweet enemy France,' crystallises that sentiment with exact felicity. For centuries France was our enemy by force of circumstance and situation; but in spite of all our wars there was always something lover-like in our feeling for that country and its radiant spirit. Even during the Napoleonic wars there was no sign of the bitterness of race hatred. When the Peace of Amiens in 1802 brought a brief interlude in warfare, all London flocked to Paris, and English travellers were greeted in Picardy with the friendliest welcome. And in 1815 when the Allied Armies marched into Paris, and Blucher, in the Prussian way we now know so well, proposed to levy a huge indemnity on the city, Wellington would not hear of it; it was not France, he said, but Napoleon, that was the conquered enemy. When the Prussians wanted to blow up the Pont de Jéna, he placed a British sentry on the bridge and defied them. Such episodes are pleasant to remember. English character is different from French character, our ways and habits of mind are equally different from theirs; but it is a difference that does not prevent a mutual admiration and respect.

On that night of the 3rd of August when, in the House of Commons, Sir Edward Grey bade us look into hearts and see if we could bear to sit with folded arms while the Germans ravaged the coasts of France, we looked into our hearts; and there were few who were doubtful of their answer. For many of us, even apart from the outrage upon Belgium, it seemed a crime beyond pardon that Germany should seek, as Germans have proclaimed, to strike down France so that she should never rise again. Take out France from the history of modern Europe, and what an inconceivable gap and loss the imagination feels! A diffusing light and energy is gone, and all our civilisation sapped and maimed. The Germans, exalting as ever their desire into fact, had repeated the creed that France was degenerate and her day of beneficence over, till they believed it. The English perhaps were too indolent and incurious to have formed an explicit opinion. They may be, they are, illogical; but of character they judge instinctively as the finger-tips of what they touch. And when they read of those interminable legions of the German army, equipped to a perfection never known before, the hugest, best disciplined and best-munitioned army ever assembled in history, launched through Belgium upon France with a momentum and velocity apparently irresistible; when they

saw with what intrepid calm and with what a noble una-
nimity the people of France turned to meet that tremendous onset; how staunchly they supported those agonising
days of suspense while the enemy each morning came ever
nearer, with so terrible a rapidity, to Paris; how they bore
the test of an abrupt and utter dislocation of their homes
and daily existence, and that perhaps still greater test, the
intoxication of victory in those miraculous September days;
– then throughout all Britain it was felt that this was a
nation by whose side we should be proud to fight, and
whose sacrifices we should be proud to share.

Nothing indeed has been more remarkable than the
unfeigned, profound, and lasting admiration of France that
her bearing in the war has evoked throughout all classes of
folk in this country, as indeed throughout the world. Of the
spontaneous sympathy with her sufferings this little record
is itself a witness; and the progressive success of France's
Day in Britain is a symptom of its deepened character.

France has not proclaimed the sufferings of her wounded
and her homeless refugees. She asked no help. What we
have done to aid her was offered simply because of our
great desire to show our loyalty and friendship, and because
of the undying debt we owe to her, not only for her Euro-
pean past, but for the unexampled burden she bore during
the first two years of this war.

Surely then, in so much common sacrifice and mutual
esteem, in admiration on either side for so vast a national
effort, there is a sure base of friendship in the future.

But this is not all. For is there any parallel in history to
the immingling for so long a period at such close quarters
of one nation with another, on terms of equal friendship,
as has happened these last years in the case of France and

England? At this moment the whole flower of our male population is abroad, and for the most part on French territory.

France, like other nations, has experienced what the sinister phrase-makers of Prussia call 'peaceful penetration.' She has experienced a foreign infiltration, professedly friendly, the extent and volume of which she never suspected till suddenly in a night she woke to find that those myriad dwellers in her cities and country towns, industrious and ingratiating, useful and well-behaved, were smiling thieves of her secrets, priers into her resources and her weaknesses returning in helmet and uniform as swaggering conquerors to the homes where they had been trusted and subservient – the implements of a patient and laborious perfidy. Nothing was further from this most odious form of German efficiency than the friendly invasion of the British soldier. Billeted in French farm and cottage, he has gone his own wonderful way, cheerfully resourceful, carrying his own world with him, little dependent on conditions, careless of the impression he makes, disguising nothing of rough exterior or natural kindness. The French peasants have come to be familiar with him, have wondered at his exuberance, his lavish washings, his light-hearted energy; they have seen him playing with their children, have noted his instinctive helpfulness and handiness.

But after all – though necessity makes itself understood easily enough – the barrier of language is a formidable one, and ignorance on either side of the other's habits and manners and ways of thought is a still greater impediment.

Take a salient instance of contrast. The French peasantry have an admirable quality of thrift. Their saving habit is no dull meanness; it is motived not only by intelligent foresight, but by devotion to their children, and often involves a long self-sacrifice. To them, the wastefulness of our soldiers in matters like cooking and feeding is something little short of monstrous; it must seem like a sort of mental vice. Waste is indeed one of our capital faults as a nation. We are as indulgent to the spendthrift's warm heart as we are indifferent to the painful lack of intelligence and proportion in our public expenditure. Yet this wastefulness belongs to qualities and energies that have made for splendour in our history. The generosity of the English people knows no limit. We are prodigals born; we like an expansive temper that enjoys the adventure of life. And to our soldiers the economical proficiency of the small French shopkeeper, for instance, still steeped in the legend that all Englishmen are rich and care nothing what they spend, is in its turn not endearing. On either side the superficial strikes more than the essential. It is useless to ignore or to lament such things. They cannot be mended by magic or in a day. Only more real and deep acquaintance can bring the larger tolerance of understanding.

No one probably can yet tell what predominant or most enduring impression will have been left by this close, yet quite unprepared-for, intermingling of two very different types of national character. Each man judges by his own temperament and inclination, within the limits of his own observation. Moreover, it is only certain parts of France which have had this experience of the English.

But in the case of our work under the Red Cross and kindred activities in France, we are on much surer ground. For here have been set up very different relations from the enforced and mostly passive acquaintance between the British Army and the French peasantry and townsfolk, where each after all has been absorbed in his own business.

In every unit there have been some, often many, who had a previous knowledge of France and of French manners and modes of thinking; who with this knowledge had a special love for the country, and who could talk to the wounded soldiers or the poor refugees in their own language. They could discuss things with them and interpret our own point of view. By the time the war is over, there will be hardly a village in France that does not contain at least one returned soldier who has known the English as friends and had familiar talk with them, in hospitals, in canteens, or at the front.

In days before hatred of England was part of the school drill of German children, Heine was eminent as a good hater of our country. He loved to contrast the stiffness of Wellington (who yet could weep tears after Waterloo because of the brave men dead) with the classic features and enchanting smile of his adored Napoleon; and he carried away from his visit to London a tourist's impression of Englishmen as all stiff, hard, and unsympathetic, each grossly immersed in his own prosaic business. But in his last years, when he lay on his 'mattress-grave' in Paris, he was visited by an Englishwoman; and, getting to know her, he came to feel that he had wronged her nation, that he had made up his mind too quickly, seen us only from the outside, and petted a prejudice that served his satiric turn. He came to believe that under the hard shell of an Englishman there might be a sound sweet kernel. So much can one drop of personal knowledge colour and change a man's conception of a nation.

Many French people before the war (like the charming and accomplished *Madame* Adam, for example) had inherited or imbibed a prejudice against Albion. But in talk with one of our English nurses, as she tends his wounds, or with one of our ladies of the canteens, as she gives him coffee and cigarettes, will not many a French soldier, if such prejudices were his, have felt them melt away? At least, when Britain is spoken of, he will have a living person to connect that name with, one who came over of her own accord to help him in his hardships and sufferings.

'Cordial Understanding' is a good word; for what is understanding without sympathy, and what is friendly feeling without understanding? To understand with goodwill; that is what we English and French need now, at this most pregnant moment of all our intertwined national history, more than anything. Just because of the absence of personal knowledge, the feeling of one country about another is little calculable and liable to strange recoils and fluctuations. And it is on this account that the work described in this little book with its resultant gradual filtering of kindly memories, its diffusion of a personal experience, of something shared in time of trouble, may prove for the future an influence much beyond the actual service rendered, and be a reassurance and a stand-by when newspapers are imagining vain things. Little rubs, resentments, and misunderstandings there will inevitably have been; there will always be these so long as human beings are human – and sometimes official. But such things are as nothing when we think of the Poilu as we have known him, and he comes before our eyes as we think of him, with his good smile, his warm grasp of the hand, his cordial, courteous, grateful speech, and his transparent friendliness. That new sense of fraternity which many in England have discovered for the first time among ourselves, of whatever class or station, is extended, for those who have worked among the French wounded and victims of the war, across the Channel. We have discovered in France, as in our own country, what wonders are hidden in the common man, what unconscious heights of heroic effort and divine self sacrifice – a finer legacy perhaps to posterity than the discovery of a superhuman genius! The stuff of our common humanity has been proved in a fiercer fire and an intenser trial than any man ever anticipated, and its worth shines out not only to confound the scoffers and scorners, but to dim the visions of dreamers.

Frenchmen and Frenchwomen, if at any time we have misinterpreted ourselves and ignorantly offended, you in your generosity will forgive; for be assured that we had no other and no greater wish than to show how Britain admired the greatness, and felt with the sufferings, of her sister nation. You did not ask for our help; but you received us as friends. What you have allowed us to do for him is little beside what we feel, now that we know him, for the simple soldier of France.

By the Same Author

POEMS OF TWO WARS
Laurence Binyon

This selection brings together for the first time the poems Laurence Binyon wrote as the world tore itself apart during two world wars, and he himself struggled to maintain a sense of goodness and hope, refusing to grow deadened to the horrors of war or to 'accept the abyss.'

ISBN: 9780993331114

Dare-Gale Press
www.daregale.com